Winning
the Chemo
Battle

Winning the Chemo Battle

❖❀❖

Joyce Slayton Mitchell

W • W • NORTON & COMPANY
New York • London

Copyright © 1988 by Joyce Slayton Mitchell
All rights reserved. Published simultaneously in Canada by Penguin Books
Canada Ltd., 2801 John Street, Markham, Ontario L3R 1B4. Printed in the
United States of America.

The text of this book is composed in Souvenir Light, with
display type set in Souvenir Demi. Composition and
manufacturing by The Haddon Craftsmen Inc.
Book design by Jacques Chazaud.

First Edition

Library of Congress Cataloging-in-Publication Data
Mitchell, Joyce Slayton.
    Winning the chemo battle.
    Includes index.
    1. Mitchell, Joyce Slayton—Health. 2. Breast—
Cancer—Patients—United States—Biography. 3.Breast—
Cancer—Chemotherapy. 4. Breast—Cancer—Psychological
aspects. I. Title
RC280.B8M556   1988   362.1'9699449[B]   87-24055

ISBN 0-393-02532-2

W. W. Norton & Company, Inc., 500 Fifth Avenue, New York, N. Y. 10110
W. W. Norton & Company Ltd., 37 Great Russell Street, London WC1B 3NU

1 2 3 4 5 6 7 8 9 0

Contents

❖❀❖

Preface

◇✿◇

Dear Reader,

Winning the Chemo Battle is a personal account of chemotherapy. If you have had chemotherapy, you will recognize the "truth" in the book, even though your own may be different. If you are about to have chemotherapy, or if a friend or relative or spouse is about to have chemo, you will get an idea of what it's like to go through this treatment by reading about someone else.

Even though this story is about one person, when we think about it, no one takes chemotherapy alone. If you have children, you will be eager to explain to them as much about cancer and crisis and death and living as well as you can. Regardless of the age of your children, you will want to reach out to them and help them understand the implications of cancer in their own family.

On the other side of you, you have parents and relatives who have had cancer or other life-threatening diseases, so when you think about where you come from, you realize the kinds of feelings and expectations that your own family history brings to you.

And then, of course, you have a spouse or good friends: your peers who want to be working this crisis out with you. They worry a lot about you, but also worry about themselves and how they would handle a life-threatening disease. Your peers wonder how they would do with a horrendous treatment like chemotherapy, as they watch you go through it.

You are not alone in chemotherapy. You bring a younger generation and an older generation and your peers with you. They all see you differently, will have needs and expectations different from yours, and will give you different kinds of support.

The goal of <u>Winning the Chemo Battle</u> is to help you plan and work toward your own quality of life. In other words, the purpose of this book is for you to see creative ways to make the best of what is . . . even with chemotherapy and the possibility of a shorter life.

Yours with hope,

Joyce Slayton Mitchell

Foreword

Jay R. Harris, M.D.

Associate Professor, Harvard Medical School
Clinical Director, Joint Center for Radiation Therapy, Boston

◇❀◇

People diagnosed with cancer have commingled fears regarding the disease and its treatment. The emotional response to the diagnosis of "cancer" is perhaps more profound than to that of any other serious illness. This is related both to the disease's potential for causing suffering and death and to its unpredictable and poorly understood behavior. Cancer is an aberration or betrayal of one's own body.

Given the consequences and fears associated with the disease, physicians and patients have been willing to treat it with strong measures that can have considerable side effects. The first efforts to cure the disease involved surgery, and this is still the major curative therapy used today. For many cancers, an adequate removal of the tumor can result in no further recurrence of the disease. Another form of local treatment is radiation therapy, used either alone or with limited surgery. Radiation therapy attempts to eradicate the tumor before it has a chance to spread. It can avoid the mutilation of radical surgery but can have various side effects. Patients diagnosed with cancer over the past fifty years have typically been confronted by the need for local treatment that is potentially disabling and mutilating.

In the past decade or so, a new method of cancer treatment has emerged. Called systemic therapy, this treatment affects the whole body, not just the local area of cancer. The most common form of systemic therapy is chemotherapy, in which chemicals are employed to kill cancer cells.

The use of systemic therapy is based on the observation that in many cases local treatment is ineffective because cancer cells have already spread through the bloodstream to others areas of the body. Systemic therapy is given either by mouth or by vein to eradicate cancer cells (or metastases) located elsewhere in the body. Chemotherapy has been shown to have significant impact on a variety of cancers.

Chemotherapy has also produced a whole new set of side effects. Patients and their family and friends need to be prepared to deal with these. In this book, Joyce Slayton Mitchell describes in a compelling and lively manner many of the typical reactions to chemotherapy and some of the coping mechanisms that were useful to her. I believe that it will help patients, their families, and their friends anticipate and cope with the effects of chemotherapy. Certainly, the personal stories will provide laughter and inspiration. I also believe that *Winning the Chemo Battle* will be useful for young health professionals (nurses and physicians) who deal with cancer patients, by helping them understand some of the emotions typical of many such patients.

A few caveats regarding the use of any lay book on cancer need to be mentioned. One is that such books should not and cannot substitute for effective communication between a patient and his or her team of health professionals. The main thrust of *Winning the Chemo Battle*—and a valuable one—is its description of the emotional response to the treatment that many people share. Moreover, because cancer and its treatment take many forms, it is neither possible nor advisable to extrapolate from one situation to another. Patients with cancer who are being treated with chemotherapy should not rely solely on the information in this book but should look for final guidance to their teams of health professionals.

Introduction

❖❀❖

October 4, 1984

Dear Ned and Elizabeth,

  I'm sorry to be writing to tell you the bad news that
you have to know. I've got breast cancer. Again. And it's
in the same place. I discovered a change in my breast
before I went to Paris, but I talked myself into thinking it
was a side effect of radiation rather than recurrent cancer.
I hate telling you about it because I hate having it.

  At least I can say that I'm glad to be writing you
now—when you are both happily at your own college,
taking courses that interest you, and are places you chose
on your own and where you are each taking so much
responsibility for financial, academic, and social areas of
your life. So at least my children are in place as I start
my second round with cancer.

I know how well you handled it when I first had cancer, five years ago. But at that time we were all living together. Now, with each of you in college in California, and your dad and I divorced and living in different places, I know a family crisis can be more confusing than ever. But do remember that we are still a family when it comes to being there for each other. You both know that, after twenty-four years of marriage, Bill and I count on each other. Our family is still a team that works together when any one of us needs unusual support.

And you both know that I have my home in place. It's the first place that's felt like home to me since I left Vermont, and I'm sure it will be a good place for healing.

And my work is certainly getting in place. Wish I could tend to a little more negotiation of book contracts before surgery. But as Dr. Samuel Hellman (same doctor I had in Boston, who has since moved to Sloan-Kettering hospital—top cancer research institute in the world, where he is physician in chief, which means the big cheese, the top dog) said to me this morning, "You can negotiate those contracts just as well November tenth as October tenth!" So—that's the end of that idea.

Now, I know that having a mother with cancer is hard on kids. Especially on you, Elizabeth, knowing a daughter's chances of breast cancer increase if her mother has it. But even increased chances don't mean you will have it. As you have both learned earlier, I know how to meet this challenge very well—and I expect the same from you.

And Ned, I realize that because of the course you took last quarter on cancer and biology, you know more about cancer than you did before, and that this makes it harder on you. The thing I learn most about—as I go along asking and reading—is that so much about cancer is unknown that it's almost impossible to predict what is going to happen with recurrence, cures, and causes. So I refuse to get scared about "what's going to happen." I'm quite sure that no one knows.

What I want each of you to do is to take this as a crisis in life and to notice how you respond to it. Whom do you tell? Whom do you not tell? What do you feel like? What do you want to ask? To know? Whom will you ask? Do you wish you knew more, knew less?

Every crisis, no matter what it is—going through a divorce, getting hurt, losing a dream, having cancer, losing a job or a friend—teaches us about ourselves and strengthens us to handle the next knock that comes our way. There isn't anyone around who doesn't get her share of crisis. If you think there is, it's only because you don't know her well enough.

Personally, I find physical knocks like cancer easier to take than relationship ones. Not that anyone has a choice: that's exactly what a crisis is—no choice—it's just thrown at you. But at least it seems the whole world is on your side with a physical illness like cancer. It's not the same with a "relationship disease" like divorce. Somehow, it's a lot easier for others to understand an illness and somehow more acceptable to be sympathetic. Even though your dad and I were miserable during the last few years of our marriage, we still respect the good years we had together and find it easier, after divorce, to be supportive of one another.

You both know that I intend to do whatever it takes to overcome this crisis, and I plan to see you both at Christmas and to come to California for your spring break, Elizabeth, and to go visit you, Ned, for your birthday in March, just the way we discussed this fall.

I think, too, that it's easier for me, the person with cancer, because I am doing something about it, than it is for the children, spouse, other relatives, and friends of the person. Even though it may be easier for me, I still expect both of you to deal with it constructively, learn and grow from it, as if it were any crisis, apply your reactions to your own life, and not use it for the things you need an excuse for. I notice I've already been tempted a couple of times to do that. For example, saying I can't do this or that because I've got cancer! Things I didn't want to do in the first place. Know what I mean?

What I would like most is for you to keep in touch with me with your letters. Nothing is a greater gift from you to me than these letters. Ned, getting your letter today just took me right out of figuring this letter out—to the enjoyment you are getting from your classes and plans for next year in Paris. And, Elizabeth, your letters to me and your artwork are always a wonderful way for us to be in touch.

I'm going to go and cook a chicken, make chicken soup, and have a nice "comfort" dinner with my friends. How I wish you two could also sit down with me and share my chicken dinner!

Courage and love,
Mom

Winning the Chemo Battle

The Chemical Takeover

◇✿◇

I was scared all right. Excited scared. The kind of scared that wonders what's going to happen next. The kind of scared that's curious. But also the protected kind of scared—within a structure that's going to take care of you. Not the being-followed-on-a-dark-street-with-no-policeman-in-sight scared.

It was 4:00 P.M. on the first day of my chemotherapy. I figured I could go right to bed and sleep for the worst of it if I made an appointment as late as possible in the day for my first chemo hit. Betsy, my tall, hardworking roommate, a health administrator, went with me. Betsy and I, both fresh from Vermont, share many friends, values, and information about each other's lives, the way old friends do. Both in our early fifties and divorced, with children in college, we form a primary support system in our New York City apartment.

We're family for each other; we appreciate each other for being there.

Betsy left work early and met me in the general waiting room on the fourth floor at the Sloan-Kettering outpatient hospital. I pretended it was nothing, like going to the dentist. I tried to appear cool, reading the *New York Times* as I figured out how to act next. An awful lot of people were there, and almost all had someone with them. Some had no hair; many were women with wigs; some read; others were visiting with their neighbors. Most were older people, a few middle-aged like me, very few young adults. The outstanding thing about the room, besides the people in it, were the exquisite flower arrangements. They reminded me of the extraordinary flowers in the Great Hall of The Metropolitan Museum. Not ordinary tulips, daffodils, and roses, they were exotic, tropical-looking flowers, three or four arranged in green bottles, in several spots around the room.

When I arrived on the fourth floor and asked for the chemo unit, I learned that I had to qualify for entry. First, I had to check in. Next, I took a number from a bakery-shop ticket machine and waited until my number was shouted over a loudspeaker so loudly that everyone in the room jumped from the jolt of the noise! Then I got to go in for a finger stick. After that, I was called to weigh in (in kilograms, which shows you how scientific they are) and to have my temperature and blood pressure measured. When I passed all of these tests (and sometimes you don't, especially on the white blood cell count), the loudspeaker again blared my name. Once more everyone in the crowded waiting room was startled by the obtrusive noise: people with hearing aids automatically reached for their volume controls. I hurried to the doctor's office. Dr. Minelli wrote my chemical prescription, and I asked him a hundred questions. He explained that he would drip (infuse slowly through a tube) an antinausea drug and give me a prescription for an antinausea suppository, which I should insert as soon as I got home. He made an appointment for a month later and sent me on to the chemo unit. I qualified. I was allowed to enter the holy of holies, the inner sanctum of the fourth floor—the chemo unit.

First I looked for a seat and place to put my coat in a very small room without windows. It was full of people whose faces expressed a little more seriousness than those did in the outer room. In this serious little room, with its few magazines, no exotic flower arrangements, a wheelchair or two hovering at the edges, I first met Connie, the chemo-unit receptionist.

I handed her my prescription, which she filed in her big black notebook. (Later I learned that when anyone forgets or loses a prescription, she always finds it in time to give the orders.) Connie is a glamorous-looking, trendy, high-fashion black woman who schedules everyone's chemotherapy. It didn't take me long to learn that she's the boss. All the chemo nurses, pharmacists, doctors, and patients go through Connie. No one gets anywhere or anything until Connie says so. Right in back of her is the open window on the pharmacy, through which she yells like a waitress to a short-order cook as she calls out, "Two Adriamycin, one Cytoxan, and three 5-FUs to go!" She knows and calls everyone by name. And she's funny.

After my first visit she asked, "How you doin'?"

"The last hit was too hard on me," I replied.

"Sorry, it must have been the wrong stuff; I'll see what I can do," was her flip response. It brought a smile to all the chemo patients, who listen to Connie for their waiting-room entertainment. When I asked her how soon I'd be called, she would go through the stacks of prescriptions, stalk out back through the chemo stations, return, and give me an accurate estimate. Connie often has candy on her desk for all of us who want it. I never once had a chemo hit without her being there. If I worked at Sloan-Kettering and had a nutrition program or a patient workshop and wanted folks to come, I'd sell her first on the program to get the people there. If I wanted to reach all of the chemo patients with a message, I'd do it through Connie. My idea of communications between hospital and patients starts with Connie. The whole Sloan-Kettering chemo unit revolves around the boss of the the chemo unit—Connie.

My first chemo nurse, Ms. Gentry, walked past Connie's desk and announced my name. She was British and the head nurse of the unit. I learned that all the nurses had special training and had received a chemotherapy certificate for this job. The unit had twenty comfortable chairs set up in private little cubbyholes. A curtain could be drawn around each chair and nurse's table, where the chemo-certified nurse always had a special platter of chemicals, designed just for me. There was a drip stand at each cubbyhole. Some chairs had one arm on them and looked like a school desk; others were like the big TV lounge chairs that many Americans buy the man in the house on Father's Day (except in sophisticated New York City, of course) or like a dentist's or barber's chair. Those lounging chairs are for the long drips, those lasting an hour or more. But my first hit, for some reason, was in a regular chair even though my drip was to last an hour. I sat right on the edge listening to every word the nurse was telling me; trying to figure out every detail that was going on. There was no way I could have relaxed and slept even if I had been in that big lounging chair! Besides, I hadn't yet learned the dangers of this nice friendly nurse and comfortable-chair chemo unit.

The nurse introduced herself; I introduced Betsy, who sat in a chair in the little cubbyhole right beside me. As it turned out, all three big hits brought a different friend into that chair. With a friend beside me, I felt as if another person's body were taking in the chemicals with me, diluting the poison so that I wouldn't get any more than I could tolerate.

The nurse started her procedure by giving me a booklet, *Chemotherapy and You: A Guide to Self-Help during Treatment,* to take home. It contained a list of chemicals and their possible side effects. She told me that chemotherapy is simply the use of drugs or medications to treat cancer. It can consist of one drug or of a group of drugs that work together. She said there are three ways to administer chemotherapy. In the oral method the drugs enter the bloodstream through the lining of the stomach or upper intestines when taken by mouth. In the intramuscular (IM) method, they are injected into a muscle in order to be slowly absorbed into the bloodstream. In the most common, the intravenous (IV, or drip), method they are injected or infused into a vein, in order to be absorbed very fast. When I jokingly said I preferred the oral, she didn't give me that choice. "How you take the drug is part of the doctor's prescription," she explained to me. "Cytoxan, for example, can be given either through a drip or orally. Chances are you will get the stronger dosage in your first three months through the drip, and the lower dosages will come later through pills you take at home."

Next, Ms. Gentry read which chemicals were prescribed for me, showed them to me in the book, and then circled each drug I was getting. At the same time, she pointed out the particular container of each chemical on her tray. First was the red syringe with the Adriamycin. Oh yes, that's the one that causes total hair loss, nausea, vomiting, lowered blood counts, red urine, and mouth sores. But the little book didn't mention the worst side effect of all, heart failure.(I knew that only because Dr. Minelli had said to me when first reviewing my record, "I'll prescribe Adriamycin if I can talk Dr. Hellman into it." "Why will you have to persuade him?"

I innocently asked. "Because one of its side effects is heart failure," he said. "Heart failure!" I shot back, "Talk *him* into it? What about me? It's my heart you're talking about!" Needless to say, he convinced us both.) The clear-looking liquid on the drip stand was Cytoxan. The list of its side effects read, "Nausea, vomiting, hair loss, lowered blood counts, blood in urine, loss of appetite." Then there was the bottle with the water "chaser" and, finally, the other syringe, containing 5-FU. I read, "Nausea, vomiting, diarrhea, lowered blood counts, mouth sores, loss of coordination, skin darkening, hair loss." The chemo nurse talked about what was going on and answered our questions the whole time I was there—just over an hour. As it was my first round of therapy, she never left my side. Ms. Gentry appeared very competent and professional, and I was as relaxed as a scared chemo patient can be. She pointed out that although some people have this or that reaction, others suffer absolutely no side effects.

After this flood of information, the first of many hunts was on for the perfect vein on the back of my right hand.

"Why do you use the back of my hand?" I asked.

"We start as far out on your extremities as possible in case the vein breaks down; then we have some place to go further up your wrist and arm. In that way, if we have to make a second puncture, the drugs won't leak from the first."

"In case the vein breaks down?" I asked.

"Yes, with continual use, especially when you're on chemo each week, the fragile veins sometimes don't hold up for carrying the drugs. Or the needle goes through the other side of the vein, and we have to find another one. We always test with water to be sure the vein will carry the drug properly."

Ms. Gentry went on, "In your case, we use only the right hand, because the lymph nodes were removed on your left side. Without a lymph system, your immune system is lowered in your left arm, and so we avoid using needles because of the possibilities of creating an infection on that side." Oh yes, I remembered that from postsurgery classes. When I made a fist while a rubber band constricted my upper arm, several good possibilities presented themselves. The first time was the best time. The experienced nurse easily found my fresh, new hand vein. One tiny prick, a piece of tape, and a lot of conversation about what she was looking for, and it was all done. She injected a shot of water into the taped needle on my hand to test her route, then proceeded to the first chemical.

Cytoxan, a clear colored liquid, dripped from a bottle hanging on the drip stand in front of me through the plastic tubing and into the needle on my hand. Ohhhhhhhhh—strange feeling in my nose—cold—the Cytoxan looks like vodka, feels like the first fresh horseradish of the season in Vermont, opening every nose and sinus passage. I can hear my father at our Easter table saying, "Good for what ails you; it clears out your head!" Only this time it won't go away! My nose feels exposed, way inside. The Adriamycin is red, like a danger sign. Will she inject it from the syringe? Why are two chemicals in syringes instead of in bottles? Oh, good: she injects it in the needle already taped to the back of my hand, and I get all four drugs in one needle. Phew. That's a help. How can people be scared of a tiny little needle when they've got a great big, life-threatening cancer and when this is the only opportunity for knocking those cancer cells dead? Easy.

For the last one, another syringe was injected, but 5-FU was a nothing experience. No color, no Cytoxan-like response in my nose and head. Nothing. Just as easy as the water chaser that hopefully cleaned out my veins, washing away the heavy chemicals. I said my thank-yous, good-byes, and that-wasn't-so-bad. Then Betsy and I left.

We splurged and took a cab home. I could have walked. But being scared cautious now, I had all antennae out to see what was going on in my body. How would I respond? Did I feel light-headed? Weak? Slowed down? Thirsty? Drowsy? Wide awake? What were those chemicals doing in my body as I walked out of Sloan-Kettering?

I felt good. Not exuberant high-energy, but good.

Several friends called when I got home by 7 P.M., and a church friend came by with Chinese take-out food for Betsy and herself, in case I had a problem with cooking smells. I started drinking my quota of water and liquids right away to flush out those killer drugs as soon as possible—as I had been told. Betsy stood close by but could see I was moving very much on my own steam, so she didn't hover. I watched Dan Rather. I was very aware of my body and was happy that I felt so good. At seven-thirty I decided to eat with my friends, mostly the bland rice. After all, I wasn't feeling a bit queasy. So we sat down, joyful that it had been so easy—nothing like what I had heard. Besides, Chinese food was my favorite. In fact, I was ravenous. By then I had decided that rice would be the perfect food to sop up all those drugs running around in my body and to diminish any possible side effects. So, I ate more than usual. And why not a few vegetables? And why not try the wonton? Everyone was in a good mood. My friends were glad that I'd accepted the chemo treatment after all and were happy with the thought that I would be getting the best cancer treatment in the world. Soon, though, I began to feel a little odd, and I was the first to leave the table. Although unable to describe what the odd feeling was exactly, I was very sure that it wasn't normal. But I was glad to feel a little sleepy. I went to bed at nine o'clock with a slight feeling of a chemical buildup—whatever that is—in my body, something like tight skin all over my body, with my flesh and liquids expanding within that skin.

I dozed off and then opened my eyes. I saw the clock. It was 11 P.M., six hours after my first hit. All of a sudden, VA VA VA VOOM! The chemical takeover: my feet hit the floor,

I bounded into the bathroom, flipped up the seat just in time to explode like a time bomb into the toilet. Betsy, whose room is closest to the bathroom, had heard me coming. Her cool hand was on my hot head, just as my mother's hand had been during all that carsickness when I was three, four, and five years old, and just as, later the hand of Bill, my former husband, had been whenever I had three martinis. But there—loving hands on my sick forehead—the similarities ended. I threw up, retched, vomited, heaved, and retched some more and just couldn't stop. My body felt bloated in every direction, my skin stretched and punctured as if I'd thrown up through each pore in my body. I couldn't stop. Every grain of rice, every sip of water, that horrendous wonton taste made me shudder to my soul, and I got sicker and sicker as I knelt there. Finally, staggering up, I reached for the green plastic basin that I'd brought home from Sloan-Kettering surgery, to take to my room. I glanced at the mirror on my way out and saw a red, puffy face with a rash just as if I had the measles. I staggered back to bed, thanking Betsy for being there.

My chemo sickness had seriously begun. I found and inserted the prescribed antinausea suppository, remembering how I'd used suppositories with both children when they were sick babies. I thought of Ned when he'd been sick from his toxic asthma medicine. I thought of my mother and her excruciating migraine headaches when I was a little girl. I thought of being in labor with both children and unable to ever get comfortable.

The antinausea stuff made me drowsy and weaker. Oh no. I could feel the buildup coming again. I tried lying on my side, my stomach, my back. Nothing worked. What was happening to me? Restless, but trying to stabilize my body with willpower, I was overcome again by the feeling of the time bomb going off as I ran down the hall to the toilet, retching for what seemed ages. Groaning, I staggered back to bed.

Oh, I thought, if only I can find a comfortable position. I feel so weak I can't relax. I don't have the strength to figure it out. I toss and turn. What's happening? I feel the buildup again. Its 1 A.M. I can't hold it in. I can't relax. I can't stabilize.

I grabbed the green basin and ran, throwing up before I got to the toilet. Oh, that rice: there's more in my stomach— those Chinese-sauce tastes repulse me. How could I have been so dumb as to eat anything? Oh Lord, let me stop retching so that I can just stand up and get back to bed.

Why isn't there relief after throwing up? Why don't I feel better? There's nothing in my stomach to come up. Why can't I find a good position in bed? Close your eyes—try to relax. How did I do it with childbirth pains? What were those relaxing exercises I learned? This is worse: there's no relaxing in between. There must be a way to let go. What is this tension, this constant buildup?" Oh no, back to the bathroom. It's 2 A.M. Betsy won't have any sleep tonight, and she needs her rest for her job.

"Betsy, how can I keep throwing up? I can't stop retching. Don't get up with me next time. Look at my skin—its so red and puffy." Ohhhhhh, get back in bed, when will it be over? Do the cancer cells feel all of this? Are they getting wiped out along with me? Why don't I feel better after I throw up? Why can't I handle this better? It's 4 A.M., then 5, 6, 7, and 8 A.M. I am throwing up on the hour. "Betsy, don't you have to go now? You've brought your work home for the morning? Oh, that's wonderful!"

How can I keep throwing up? I've used these suppositories every four hours. They seem to make me weak and just as nauseous. Not again! At 9 A.M. a shorter retching; another at 10 A.M. Will it ever stop? 11 A.M.; I'll just stay here. I'm not going into the bathroom again. I can't make it again. I'm practically crawling back to bed. Betsy even has to take my arm. I'm absolutely exhausted. What do people do who are alone with this? I'll close my eyes; I don't feel the buildup. My stomach is so sore. I'm so hot, I'm so miserable. I drift off. It's been twelve hours. Oh, thank you, God, P-E-A-C-E at last. I hear Betsy on the phone: "Hard night—she's resting" I quickly snatch my green basin: just a little spit. It's over. Chemo Hit No. 1.

Thank God for Betsy. We came to share an apartment because she came down from Vermont a year after me to take on the biggest private home health agency in the country, as vice-president of New York City's Visiting Nurses Service. But before all of that she herself was a nurse. She's my resource for figuring everything out, my primary source of medical information. "What is this drug, and what is that? What does Cytoxan do? Have you heard of 5-FU? Will you find out about Adriamycin? Does it really hurt your heart? Why do I crave sugar? Why is my face red? Why is my whole body hot? How can you stand these chemical smells in our apartment? Did Bill, Elizabeth, Ned call? What did you tell them? Do we have any apples? Or canned fruit? Who's in the living room? What time is it? Do you think ginger ale would be good for me? Oh, Betsy, thank you for holding my head! Can you close my window? The chemical smells are still coming in! What time will you be home? What is Methotrexate? Cytoxan? Is Prednisone the same thing used for tennis elbow? What's the difference between dripping in Cytoxan and taking it orally? Why can't everything be oral? Can you imagine, Betsy, they prescribed an oral antinausea when they know I can't stop throwing up? Is it hot in here? Is it cold in here? Do we have any potatoes, pasta, oatmeal? Are there any visiting nurses who teach relaxation techniques? Are there any nutrition nurses especially for cancer? I know the VNS has the best hospice program in the Big Apple, but I hope I'm not yet ready to ask for that!"

I'm so weak my stomach hurts. How can I recover? The

sooner I get some food in my stomach, the sooner I'll be able to stabilize. I sleep an hour, then another hour. My clock reads 1 P.M. and then 2. Then it's 5 P.M. Twenty-four hours have passed since my hit. Oh, I'm so weak and miserable. Maybe a little banana will help. That's what they feed sick babies in New Guinea: ripe banana, easy on the stomach. Oh, it's so sore. I'm so thirsty. I can't possibly drink anything and won't be able to flush out those chemicals in my bladder, my liver, my kidneys, and where else did they say? Oh, God.

It's now been forty-eight hours. Maybe an ounce of ginger ale. When Ned was a little boy and taking powerful medicine, his doctor said, "Just an ounce of liquid to see if it stays down." Oh, Ned, I never realized how your body felt on that asthma medicine every four hours for years. Did I comfort you enough? Is this how you felt? Was I patient with you? Oh, God, that tastes good. Feels as if I could drink two ounces. Better not.

Two and a half days after my first hit. Oatmeal. That's what I want. Oatmeal will be perfect. I remember how good that oatmeal was every Vermont winter morning. My dad always made the oatmeal. He had more ideas about how to make perfect oatmeal. I don't remember ever meeting any-one else so into oatmeal. Just before he went to bed, he would fix the oatmeal in the double boiler and set it on the register of our coal furnace. Even when the furnace was turned down as far as possible, enough heat came out of the register to cook the cereal. I'd be the first one up, and I remember that thick crust on top of the pot: I'd roll it back, putting my spoon underneath to dish out the soft part so as not to get any of the top crust. We even had a special way to eat it, learned from my grandfather. First, put the oatmeal into the hot bowl. Then make a little well in the center and fill it with maple syrup. Next, pour heavy cream (of course nowadays I use milk) on the outside edge of the dish, just enough so it doesn't go over the top of the oatmeal and touch the syrup. If the consistency of the oatmeal is perfect, it floats in the milk and swirls all in one piece in the bowl. Finally, with the first bite make a little channel between the maple syrup and the milk and let the milk flow in the center, while the syrup flows out. I can just see it now. Oh boy! I'm going to survive this inhumane treatment. Hmmmmm. Oatmeal.

Cancer Is
a Family Affair

❖❀❖

Cancer, of course, doesn't begin with chemotherapy. When you get cancer, or when family or friends get cancer, it helps to think through where you and they are coming from. What is your family experience with this life-threatening disease? What is your family history with cancer and chemo? What are your perceptions of cancer, or of people with cancer? What do you say to yourself about cancer in general? The kinds of help you need and offer others depend very much on where you are. How do you cope with crisis in general? With a health crisis in particular? With injustice, with learning that the world's not fair, with terribly bad luck?

It's no wonder that although I now lived in New York, I thought only of going to Boston to check out my cancer. After all, I have a family history of cancer and of going to

Boston to do something about it. Even my grandfather, who earned his living hunting foxes during the Great Depression in northern Vermont, ended up in Boston for his cancer treatment.

When I first got cancer, I realized what a unique example I had to follow. In 1974, just five years before I was diagnosed for the first time, my dad had died of the disease. But he didn't die without being very aware that he was living through his last year and enjoying every single minute of it. At the time I was married and living in Vermont. My husband, Bill, and I and two children had just returned from a two-year anthropological expedition in New Guinea when my dad finally checked out his hunch that he had cancer. I remember my dad's operation in the early spring, followed by his "last trout season." In the fall came his "last patridge season," when the Mitchells went to Hardwick for Sunday dinner. My mother cooked his hunt to make a "patridge pie," as we Vermonters call it. Deer season, in late November, got a little tough, as my dad was much frailer, even though he drove out to our farm in his special hunting car.

His Model A Ford was rebuilt with modern brakes and was, according to him, better than any modern four-wheel drive for Vermont back roads. I remember driving to so many early-morning deer stands in that car. As a small ten-year-old with my own gun, I was squeezed in the backseat between Bob White, the famous basketball coach from St. Albans, and Archie Post, the track coach at the University of Vermont. That Model A was alive with hope, excitement, and expectation of a big buck bounding out of the woods, as we bumped along those frozen, washboard Vermont back roads clad in our red-and-black hunting wools. We stopped at the fresh deer tracks around an apple orchard to take our stand just before sunrise.

On this hunting day my dad stood on our porch waiting for Bill to go with him, holding that heavy deer rifle with a scope, hardly able to breathe, because his emphysema was getting worse. But able to breathe and walk or not, George Dix Slayton got in his "last deer season."

When my dad appeared to be in his very last days, he asked my mother to invite all the relatives for a last meal together. He had a very bad night, and my mother kept hoping he would tell her to call it off. Finally, at 5:30 A.M., he asked her to come closer so that she could hear him. Thinking he had changed his mind about the dinner, she moved closer and just barely heard him whisper, "Sally, when you cook the duck, be sure you put just a little tiny bit of garlic under the wing." My mother said to me later, "All this time I thought he was lying awake worried about how long the cancer would go on, what would it be like to die, how much worse would he get; when all the time he was lying there thinking of that wonderful duck dinner at his family table."

The best thing about my dad's last year was that he had no regrets. He planned to live until he was seventy, and he died when he wanted to—two days after his birthday. He never had any drugs or life-saving equipment in the small, rural hospital, to which he wouldn't go until the day before his birthday. He didn't miss a meal. He had his oatmeal in the morning, went into a coma after sending the nurses scurrying all over the hospital looking for a toothpick, and died with my mother and me in the room, right beside him, a few hours later.

He never gave up, and he never gave in. His wife and children never did get the last word. Cancer in my family doesn't change things.

That's where I come from. Living in character with cancer. I'm on solid ground. I know now, from my family heritage, that cancer patients can be more than survivors; we can be thrivers, even with recurrent cancer and chemotherapy.

True, seventy seems a lot older to me than forty-five, the age at which I first got cancer. And I didn't have a chemo model. Still, the principle is the same for all of us—to make the decision to live a quality life, whether it's one year more or thirty years more. If you know someone who has gone before you to show you the way, it helps. If you hear or read of someone who is planning his or her agenda as cancer progresses in his life, that helps, too.

If you have children, you will want to be a good model for them in your cancer crisis. Another chemo patient, a woman, said to me that her thirty-year-old daughter was scared her mother was going to die. The mother told me she had to prove to her daughter that she wouldn't die. She was shocked when I suggested that they could talk about that possibility.

I learned later from my son that, like my dad, I had been a good model for my children in 1979. It was in deer season when I left home to be treated at the Harvard Medical School radiation program in Boston. I spent six weeks there, returning to Vermont for weekends. My children were thirteen and fourteen. After Ned had taken a college course in the biology of cancer several years later, he told me, "You and dad certainly handled it well. We had no sense of losing our family."

Bill and I spent a lot of time thinking through how to deal with the children, what their life would be like at home all week, how much time he could spend there, and to what extent they could take over the cooking and home responsibilities that they usually shared with us. They both told me later that they had read John Travolta's book, *John and Diana: A Love Story,* about his lover, the actress Diana Hyland, who died of cancer. That's where they, as teenagers, got their written information about the disease!

It's easier to win the chemo battle if you begin by figuring out where you've come from with cancer and with crisis in your family. In that way you'll have a better sense of the possible directions you are likely to go. The more you know about where you come from, the better your chances of changing where you can go.

The Boston Trip

◇✿◇

Chemotherapy started for me in the fall of 1984. It all began when I innocently headed for Boston. At that time I really had no idea that I was heading for a second fight with cancer. Little did I know that my Boston trip would lead to surgery and that the surgery would lead to a long, hard haul of chemotherapy.

I couldn't put it off any longer. It was time to check out this funny-looking, electrified-feeling left breast. After all, I thought finding out didn't mean I had to do something about it right away. I thought I could wait until Elizabeth had had a good first-year start in college, Ned was solidly involved with his second college year, and I had sold one or two more book ideas—wait until everything was in place—then I would deal with cancer. If cancer had really come back.

I called Dr. Jay R. Harris in Boston. He's the physician

who, along with Dr. Sam Hellman, treated me with a six-week radiation program for breast cancer in 1979. We like each other. I love seeing his face, hearing his laugh, watching his smiling, warm, brown eyes. I explained to Jay on the phone that my left breast looked funny: it had a dividing line, a depressed nipple, and, besides that, I had had electrical-like flashes through my breast for months. I asked him if it could be a late side effect of the radiation.

Until that moment I must have been playing a strong denial game with myself all those months. I didn't have any idea how scared I was until I got on the phone. My quavering voice was a dead giveaway. As my voice let me down, I realized even more that I didn't want anything to do with recurrent cancer. I didn't want to think about it, didn't want to plan how to deal with it, didn't want to pay for it in money or in time. I was just getting started on a new life without husband and children in New York City. Even though divorce was my choice and living in the Big Apple my dream, I already had a very full agenda dealing with the difficult changes I was going through after twenty-four years on a Vermont farm with my family. Besides all of that, being divorced and self-employed, I had a minimum of health insurance and no major medical, because the cost and conditions were so high. For example, I paid about $800 a year for independent Blue Cross, and if I, with a previous cancer record, had wanted major medical it would have cost another $250 a year. There was also a $500 deductible each year. That means I would have paid $750 a year before Blue Cross paid on my major medical bills, bringing me quickly to over $1,500 a year just for the insurance.

To my telephone description, Jay immediately responded, "When can you come? Shall I line up a surgeon to see you at the same time?" I remember asking why. The suggestion of a surgeon both surprised and frightened me. I admit it now and have learned it well: denial is one of my strongest traits. After falling apart on the phone, I found it easy to agree on an early-morning mammogram appointment so that I could hand carry the results to my meeting with Jay at Boston's Beth Israel hospital.

I wrote my Boston friend Marylynn that I'd like to come and stay with her and have my friends Pat and Ellen for dinner the evening before my appointment. We decided to go out to a cheap, good health-food-type restaurant in Cambridge where we'd all been before. Three out of four of us are always strapped for money, since two of us are recently divorced and Pat is a poorly paid minister married to another poorly paid minister. We carefully choose our eating places; even more often, Marylynn or I cook at her place. We love to get together; it is never often enough. Maybe three times a year, or four at most. We always have a lively discussion about the family, women, our children in college, making money, and all the other issues that seem to crop up in middle age. We have known one another for more than twenty years and we are extraordinarily loving and accepting of each other. Our life experiences, like those of any group of three or four people, are different, but we find a lot of common ground. I consider these friends my Boston family—my Boston support group.

People Express flew me safely to Boston. I met everybody at the Cambridge restaurant and told them a lot more about my New York City struggles as a single woman than about my cancer struggles. After all, I'd been to Boston for all of my radiation follow-up visits five years earlier. My friends had met Jay Harris when I was being treated, and they had even called him when other friends or clients or parishioners were in cancer trouble. My friends have counted on Dr. Harris because he has always taken the time to answer their questions and concerns. One New York friend even carries Jay's name and phone number with him and has had worried friends call him from all over the country. No one thought it unusual for me to be in Boston with an early-morning appointment with Jay.

I kept my mammogram appointment at 8:00 A.M., even though I had sworn I would never have another one. My first mammogram, five years before in Vermont, and a second in Boston under the direction of the Harvard Medical School both turned out to show no cancer, when, in fact, my lump was malignant. To say that, after that experience, I was reluctant to agree to an annual mammogram is an understatement. However, Drs. Hellman and Harris convinced me that they needed a "baseline" record from which to judge changes in the future. "It is," they said, "good scientific medicine." As I knew my insurance covered only half the cost of a mammogram, it took a lot of convincing. I had no interest in spending my hard-earned and hard-saved money on something that didn't work and that, even worse, was so misleading to me.

I sat up on the edge of the examining table, with its freshly rolled-out paper, and chatted with Jay about our jogging schedules, careers, and children. Finally, we turned our attention to my problem: depressed nipple, divided breast, electrical-like waves through the months of April, May, June, and July. I hadn't looked at my breast in the month of August, because I'd been in Paris and the mirror in my rented apartment there was too high.

"Jay, do you suppose my condition could be a side effect of radiation?"

"Five years after? Unlikely. We need a biopsy right away, I'll go and call Dr. Bradley while you're still here. You'll like him. He likes to answer questions, and I'm sure he'll consider your ideas in his decisions."

"Well, wait a minute. I can't have breast cancer without a lump, can I?" Oh-oh, there's that quavering voice of mine again.

Jay nods.

With steady voice once again, because of a sudden, inspirational optimism, I ask, "But where would you take the biopsy if there isn't a lump?"

Jay points and says, "There. Or there. Or there or there."

"What if it's cancer, can I be radiated again?"

Jay shakes his head.

"Surgery?"

The nod is affirmative.

I'm feeling a little scared. But not too scared. After all, it's probably not really cancer. No one knows without a biopsy.

Jay and I looked at my mammogram together, saw nothing, and looked at the previous one. Then Jay said, "We can't really compare them, because we've got a new machine which is much finer, but it means that comparisons aren't valid." That's it! Never again, even for so-called scientific baseline data or for whatever medical reasons, am I going to pay for another mammogram. NOT EVER! Maybe they help others, but mammograms have never added accurate information to my medical record.

I went to meet the new doctor, whose office was just a few blocks from Beth Israel. Jay had called to set up the appointment for me. The outstanding thing about the surgeon was his good looks. He was tall, had gray hair and plenty of it, a great smile, and great teeth, and wore a pinstripe suit. To me he looked more expensive Wall Street than academic medical world. When Dr. Bradley told me he had been in the same medical school class as Sam Hellman, who he knew had treated me, the thought raced through my mind that it must have been a very competitive year, so the admissions committee added "tall, dark, and handsome" to the usual academic criteria for that medical school class.

The surgeon was as friendly as he was good-looking. We talked a while; I think he mentioned that if he found a malignancy, a mastectomy would be my only choice at that point. When I said I wasn't quite ready for that surgery, he agreed that it wouldn't make that much difference if it were done within the month. His son had just been married in Vermont, he skied in Vermont, he loved Vermont. Our deal was made: a biopsy with local anesthesia for 8 A.M. the following day.

Neil, Marylynn's first-year-medical-student son, was studying when I returned to the apartment and announced that I'd be staying overnight after all, for an 8:00 A.M. biopsy. Searching my face for clues about how I was taking this pronouncement and not quite sure how to respond, Neil expressed great warmth and empathy as he said he was sorry to hear that a biopsy was necessary.

I was eager to get busy cooking dinner for the three of us. I was counting on my usual broken-heart exercise—cooking —to stabilize and calm me. I began to cut the vegetables while drinking a beer. Then I warmed the pan and added parsley and garlic to the butter and set the table. I moved quickly and confidently around the kitchen, determined to shut out broken-heart feelings.

If you've been in this situation, you'll remember that once the possibility of having cancer hits you, a jumble of thoughts race through your head: Loss of good health, death, vigilance, early death, courage. Do I have cancer? What if I do? When will I tell anyone? When will I tell my children? Ned is in Vermont this weekend coming through New York City for a day or two on his way to Santa Cruz; how can I not tell him? Think of the sympathy I'll get. Everyone will say, "Oh no, not again! You don't deserve this." As if the world were just and people got what they deserve. "You're so strong. I would never handle it that well." Drama. Excitement. Focus on my cancer life, focus off divorce, off New York City, off selling and writing books, off making a living, off figuring out how to live as a divorced woman, off finding family and community in my friends and church. Focus completely on getting rid of cancer, doctors, hospital appointments—on healing. If I have cancer again, I know I'll free myself from everything else in order to concentrate my entirety on healing. Deep, deep, deep down, what do I really think? Do I have cancer? No, I have to say, I honestly don't know.

I had planned to take Boston's "T," the subway-trolley, from Cambridge to Beth Israel for my early-morning biopsy. After all, I knew well how to get to cancer-cure places in Boston. I'd been there before: every day for six weeks five years earlier. But Marylynn wanted to drive me to Beth Israel.

She had inherited her old car when her mother died several years earlier. There was a child's safety seat in the back, a dented fender, and a broken window. That car was a dramatic symbol to me of the feminization of poverty—of women's living conditions after divorce. The notion of Bill or Hal, our former husbands, driving up to a hospital for a cancer biopsy in that wreck of a car was ludicrous. I thought of Hal, who now owns a new Mercedes, and of Bill, with his brand-new Mercury wagon, which would have been driven by their live-in girlfriends. The image was so different from the reality of the two of us in that beat-up old car that I almost forgot where I was going! Marylynn offered me what she had: a couch in the two-bedroom apartment she was sharing with her son. She wanted me to be sure to know that I could stay there after surgery in order to be in Boston for my follow-up visits. There we were: both over fifty, each with a liberal arts degree, plus a master's degree, bright, from good homes, wives for more than twenty-four years, homemakers until our children had left. We were just what the 1950s had taught us to be. Oh Lord, look at us now. Don't miss this beat-up old car, Lord. And our tiny, rented apartments, while our old husbands own our family homes. Pure social injustice. Maybe just a little of that social injustice could be traded off for some healing. Lord?

Marylynn gave me several phone numbers where I could reach her all day and asked me to be sure and call if I needed her or wanted a ride to the airport or to stay over another night. Even though I walked in on my own, I was very much aware that I was not alone; I knew I had a loving friend a phone call away.

I checked in with a cheerful young nurse. I knew the system—this was my second biopsy under local anesthesia. I didn't want to ride up to the operating room (OR) on a wheeled bed, as if I were sick. After all, when you go to the dentist, you don't get treated as if you couldn't walk. That handsome Dr. Bradley came dashing in and said I could go up in the elevator with him. I walked in and hopped up on the OR table. He told several one-liner jokes, and I laughed. He sang a few lines from several songs, "Life Is Just a Bowl of Cherries," "I've Got the World on a String," and "Mares Eat Oats," as he began his procedure. I am always glad when the doctor checks out which breast we are talking about, even though it looks so obvious. He introduced me to the nurses in the room and told me they were going to clean and swab the area with something that looked like iodine. Next, a local anesthesia was given, just like a shot of novocaine at the dentist's. A sheet was put between my eyes and the biopsy area, so I couldn't see what was going on. I'm happy to say that I couldn't feel what was going on either. But I could feel a tugging and pressure where he was cutting, so I knew when he was between cuts. After he had been working and singing away jovially for about fifteen minutes, I asked, "How does it look in there?"

"Like a radiated breast. . . . I've never seen anything that looks quite like this." Oh-oh, I thought. That's it. Well, maybe not. Lets see. It's Wednesday. Lab tests will take until Friday. When on Friday? What if he calls and I'm not home? What if my answering machine doesn't work? What will the weekend be like if I have to wait till Monday to hear the results?

While he sang and whistled away, I continued through my series of what-ifs.

Finally I peppered him with questions: "What time of day do you usually get the results? What time of day do you usually call? I want to be sure and be there when you call. Will I know before the weekend?" He replied slowly, "Just a minute here," while keeping his head down and concentrating on the task. "Let's see. . . . I'm about done here. You may not like what I find, but I think I may be able to tell you before you leave. . . ."

No more jokes. No more songs.

Oh no, I thought. But then I remembered it takes a biopsy to know.

"You get dressed and don't leave," he said. "I'll meet you downstairs. I think I'll have an answer for you."

Wheeled out of the OR and downstairs, I hopped off the moving bed and looked in the mirror. I saw myself in a blood-stained white gown, operating cap, thickly bandaged chest, and those funny-looking, way too big, disposable slippers. I looked at myself—and looked some more. I looked straight into my eyes and asked, "Do you have cancer?"

"I don't know."

In the mirror I saw Dr. Bradley rushing in before I'd even had time to dress—that was fast!

"Here," he said, "let's sit down. When a surgeon pulls up a chair, you've got to watch out." I sat down.

"You've got cancer," he told me.

"Same as before?"

"I don't know. We have to check that out with your last slides."

"What's next?"

"You may remember me saying yesterday that a mastectomy is the only choice. We won't know how extensive it is until we know more about lymph node involvement and the particular cancer."

"Is time important?"

"I'll go along with you and say anytime in the next month, the sooner the better."

"Okay, I'll think about it and be in touch with you."

"Any other questions?"

"No."

I got dressed, very slowly. The bad news was sinking in. I knew it now. "I've got cancer. Again. Same place," I told the cheerful nurse.

How come I know I have cancer again? I wasn't supposed to hear until the end of the week. In my own apartment. With my friends nearby. What am I doing here alone with this bad news? No tears came. No gripping fear—just slowed way down. Got to get this zipper up, my beads on. My bandage doesn't look bad, no throbbing underneath yet. Got to get back home. My God, I've got cancer!

Karen will come over. She told me to be sure and call if I wanted someone to talk anytime I got back to New York. She takes a late lunch, so I had a new goal: to be in the city by one o'clock. My whole life centered on that goal. I focused all of my energy on my goal of reaching New York City by one o'clock. I could talk it over with her in my own apartment. I hurried on. Betsy can be home by seven if I call her when I get in.

I'll splurge on a cab to take me to the Longwood trolley, which will get me to the Boston airport. I feel a little light-headed. Don't see a cab, nice clear day, will walk slowly down Longwood toward the trolley, and get a cab on the way. . . . God! I'm almost there. Imagine walking out of here. With cancer. By myself! To this trolley two miles away. I wasn't supposed to know today I had cancer. Jesus! No seats on the trolley. Don't I look disabled? Holding my left hand up, with all of these bandages. God! I guess not. No one is budging. Interesting, I must look ordinary. Get to the airport, glad my bag is light, get right on People, not thinking much, just have to move slowly and surely, straight toward New York City. One straight line. One direct goal. Home. Somehow I'm on the plane, no tears, all business. I have cancer. When will I deal with it? Can I morally keep it from Ned and Elizabeth? Can I morally tell others that I have cancer before I know what I'm going to do about it? Wouldn't they feel they had to convince me to move on it, considering how the world views cancer? I'm in Newark now, on the bus to the Port Authority Terminal. It's only 12:30. Home by 1:00.

"Hi, Karen, this is Joyce. I made it by 1:00! Can you come over for lunch? I've got my biopsy results. . . . Your office is too busy? Yeah, but . . . you said. Oh. I see. Well, after work, then? At 5:30? You've got cocktails at 5:30? Karen, I really need to be with a friend. He's from out of town? After your class at 8:30? Oh."

WHAM! My moment of truth. I put the receiver down. It hits me full force. I'm alone. No friend to distract me. No lunch to cry through. No great plan of action to work out with a friend. No alternative to explore with another person. No hand to hold. No theories to voice. Just me. Just me, Oh Lord. Standing before you in great need. Oh Lord, I've got cancer, what are we going to do about it?

The easiest thing to do was to feel very very very sorry for myself. I called Betsy and told her, "I've got cancer."

"Oh God! Shall I come right home?"

"No. I'll be okay. I'll take a nap and cook. Can you come at six?"

"Sure."

Ned called. He has changed his plans and will be in New York City tomorrow night and leave early the following morning for California. Is that okay? It's wonderful for me. I can't wait to see my son. I'll wear a loose shirt over this bulky bandage.

Bill was the only one in Vermont who knew about the biopsy. The best thing we, like many divorced couples, do together is parenting, and cancer for me seemed like a parenting issue. Chemo would soon become a parenting issue, too. I didn't want to tell other relatives and then have to worry that Ned and Elizabeth would hear the news from someone else. And I wanted to tell them after I decided what I was going to do about it and when I was going to do it. Thinking through my next steps, I was presented with still another solution at dinner: Betsy in her quiet, managerial voice asked whether I'd considered having surgery in New York City. She went on, "Sam Hellman is here, Sloan-Kettering is nearby. You could walk there for follow-up and any further treatment you may need. You would be home for recovery and follow-up. If it turns out you need chemotherapy, you'd be nearby. . . ."

"New York? Of course not! Vermonters go to Boston in a medical crisis. . . . I go to Boston for cancer. Besides, that's where I went before, and I know where everything is: Sydney Farber Cancer Institute, the Deaconess Hospital, the Deaconess Radiation Center, Beth Israel, Longwood Avenue subway stop, Marylynn's apartment, the Deaconess Coffee Shop's grilled cheese sandwiches I love, and the mailbox just outside the door where I always post my letters describing my latest cancer adventures. And the same doorman who's been there for years and is always so friendly, the cafeteria around the corner, the deli around the other way, Joslin Park and benches where I can picnic when it's nice outdoors. All of those important things."

Betsy didn't say anything. I thought about what she said. And thought some more. It made sense. Why hadn't I thought of it? Of course, I'll go to Sloan-Kettering. It's the most famous cancer center in the whole wide world. Besides, Sam Hellman is there, and I can walk there. And I'll be at home. With my word processor and my work and my friends and my church. "Why, Betsy, what a good idea!"

I called Dr. Samuel Hellman. When we met, several years after he had treated me in Boston, I felt as if I were back in familiar territory, on safe ground. A physician I trusted, he is about my age and has dark curly hair, an engaging laugh, and blue eyes, as well as the best taste in perfectly fitted wool suits I've ever seen. He told me that I'd been procrastinating. He called in Dr. H. M. Sockol. I was scheduled for a modified radical mastectomy one week later. Chemotherapy was on its way.

Notes from the Floor: Memorial Sloan-Kettering

❖❀❖

I never think of myself as a loner. And yet, it turns out that I do a lot of things alone that others do with some-one. Like entering Memorial Sloan-Kettering alone for surgery.

Most chemotherapy patients start out as surgery or radia-tion patients. Those in surgery face a relatively brief hospital stay when the tumor is removed and the extent of the cancer is determined. At that time they learn the recommendations for follow-up. Increasingly, the follow-up treatment is che-motherapy.

I'll never forget finding out about the surgery part of this chemo ordeal. When Dr. Hellman called in a surgeon, I had to face the tough questions that many of you will recognize: How do you feel when you don't like your doctor? What do you do when the doctor you've been told is "wonderful," "tops in the field," "the only one to go to" turns out in your first encounter to be everything that doesn't work for you? You can read about how to choose a doctor, and you can get evaluation lists and recommendations from the American Cancer Society and cancer hospitals and the National Cancer Institute, but what are you going to do when your doctor treats you as if you couldn't possibly understand what this disease is going to do to you? How do you feel at age fifty when he calls you Mary, or John, and you can't even find out his first name and are expected to respond to a thirty-year-old, to one the age of your daughter or son, with "Yes, Dr. Sockol"? What's it like for you when the doctor pats you on the cheek or the back and says, "Now just don't worry about that question," or, even worse, when a confrontation is the beginning of your relationship?

Dr. Sockol, who was very European with his perfectly manicured red beard, was the surgeon recruited for me by Dr. Hellman. Our first encounter had ended in a shouting match when he yelled, "If you'd had surgery in the first place, you wouldn't be in this mess, but, oh no, you wanted to conserve that breast, didn't you, and it didn't work, did it?"

I shouted back, "Would you like to repeat that to your radiologist boss, Sam Hellman, who prescribed my breast radiation treatment and to whom you report?" He rose to the top of his toes at full height of six feet two or three, closed his eyes, and in his best Eastern European accent warned, "You don't seem to understand the gravity of this situation." Then he turned on his heel and walked out!

Jesus! I knew surgeons were arrogant, but did I want to be asleep under his knife? This confrontation had started when he began to describe what he was going to cut away. I asked him how he knew what he was going to do before he had learned where the cancer was. When I said I wanted to be sure to end up with the use of my left arm, he snapped back, "What do you need that for? Are you a typist or something?" God! I need my left arm for a lot of things!

As soon as I got home, I called Sam Hellman and asked him if he owed Dr. Sockol a favor and if that was why he brought this particular surgeon in for me. He laughed and said, "No, he's the best there is. You aren't going to him for his TLC; you need him for his surgical skills. Besides that, he'll be easier to meet the second time."

"But where will I get my TLC?

"From me."

Relief! Okay, I'll call Dr. Sockol and see him once more before surgery. I can't afford not to.

Trying hard to restore perspective after our first meeting, we talked about fifteen minutes. He asked whether I had relatives who'd had cancer. He drew a diagram as I answered that my mother's sister died of cancer and that her niece, my cousin, had breast cancer. Then he asked, "No cancer on your father's side?"

"Yes, my dad died of cancer. But I didn't mention it, because five years ago, they just wanted to know my mother's side."

"Well, we've found new evidence that links the father's side to breast cancer. I hope he didn't have cancer of the colon."

"He did."

"Look at this diagram. You're in the cross fire from all sides of your family, aren't you?"

"Yeah."

"Okay, we agree that I take out everything I see and no more than is necessary for your particular situation. You know I'll be in San Francisco for a medical meeting after Thursday, and someone else will follow up. You're from Vermont? I'm taking my family there to ski this winter. It's a beautiful place."

Dr. Hellman was right. Our second meeting was better.

The problem when we don't like our doctor is that we want to ask our questions but don't want to upset "the doctor." It's scary. We don't like to think of the consequences if the doctor doesn't like us. We want answers and we want technical skill, but we want, too, to have a warm, friendly person there, relating to our stress and worry with this life-threatening disease with so many unknowns. Once we've checked out the qualifications of a doctor and learned that he or she is connected with a hospital, has specialized in cancer (oncology), is recommended by a medical group, and seems to have the right credentials, then we have to ask ourselves, How important is it to like this doctor, to get along with him or her? After all, we're grown-ups. We have learned by now that life isn't ideal: we can't always find the friendly, skilled doctor we wish were treating us. I think most of us will go for the credentials, as documented by the doctor's hospital affiliation, and work at the personal aspects. It takes the same friendship skills to get along with a doctor as with anyone else, except that usually the balance of power between patient and doctor falls heavily on the doctor's side. It's even worse when it's a female patient and a male doctor. Trying to be assertive by being honest and open and willing to keep trying to communicate is the best way to right the balance. Learning how to deal with doctors who are too busy to talk, cold, patronizing, and abrasive is usually worth the effort. In other words, don't let their offensive behavior frighten you into not trying for a better relationship. Of course, they won't all be bad. Many of you will also have found a competent, friendly Jay Harris or Sam Hellman in your medical saga.

After it was decided that I'd be admitted for a modified radical mastectomy, I was told that I'd be called by 9:00 A.M. on Monday, Tuesday, Wednesday, or Thursday to be admitted by noon of that day. In other words, I was to be packed to go Monday through Thursday. Almost no one outside of New York City can believe that this is standard procedure for admission. Sloan-Kettering is so crowded, there is such a long waiting list, there are so few surgical slots to be filled in the operating room that each new patient gets in line each week for admission. Of course, I wanted to know what my chances were for the first, second, third, or fourth day. How could I let Bill know when to come down if I didn't even know until three hours before? Besides that, what would I do Monday, Tuesday, or Wednesday after learning I wasn't going in? What do other people do who have left their jobs and are just sitting around and waiting to be admitted? How do mothers of young children work it out with their families? Do they tell their kids that "maybe" their mommy will go to the hospital today? What do rigid people do with this system, or frightfully scared people? Isn't it kind of inhumane? A kind of torture?

I believed, though, in the it-won't-happen-to-me theory. I also figured I had other things going for me: Dr. Hellman's name was on my record, I was a recurrent case, and everyone at Sloan-Kettering had decided I had procrastinated enough. And so I thought my chances of admission on the first day would be great. They were.

At noon I purposefully walked to the hospital, just about a mile away from my apartment, and found an unusually attractive admitting office, with paintings on the wall and cut flowers on the desk. Once I was in admissions, the excitement started to build: I panicked only once, when my insurance was checked.

I thought, Oh my God, they'll find out I don't have enough insurance and won't take me after all of this. I should never have gotten divorced and lost out on Bill's 100 percent insurance coverage. I beat the Russian roulette admissions system for Monday, Tuesday, Wednesday, or Thursday, and now I won't be let in, because I can't pay. Whom can I call? What can I say? But, no, she smiled and said, "Your Blue Cross is all in order." Phew.

As if in a hotel, I was told the room was not ready yet, and I was to wait in the waiting room on the eighteenth floor. The eighteenth . . . Wow! Hotels with a view cost more! Great view, wonderful light.

Of course, it didn't take too long to find out that Sloan-Kettering eighteen also means breast cancer, no "view" or "cost" factor in it.

Walking in to the smoke-filled waiting room was my first problem. I refuse to be understanding about how a hospital can assign cancer patients to a smoke-filled area, no matter what the rationale. I think it's absoluteley immoral. I remembered my outrage at Boston's Sydney Farber Cancer Institute, where they also had a smoke-filled lobby for cancer patients in which I once had to wait for radiation measurements. This time I found a wheelchair in the hall to sit in. As I sat there, I calmed down from the injustice of smoke; from the injustice of getting cancer again; from the injustice of getting cancer in the first place; from the injustice of being divorced; from the injustice of still being so poor in spite of all the books I'd published. All those injustices of life came rolling around my body and swirling through my mind in that smoke-filled-room assignment.

If you've ever gone to the hospital for surgery, you'll remember what your room was like. Did it have a TV, a phone, a view, a roommate or two? Was it big or tiny? Did it have windows looking out to anything? Did it smell like a hospital? My aunt Eunice is always wanting to give me something or do things for me. Before I went into the hospital, I told her I'd love to have a phone and a TV while I was there if she'd like to pay for these extras for me. But when I got to my room I learned those two things were part of the package. They come automatically with the eighteenth floor. The little TV was about four by six inches and came down by the bed on an arm, just like a study lamp. Pretty nice place.

Going to new places, even to a hospital, teaches us a lot about who we are. Have you noticed how excited you get when you pack for the hospital? Is that excitement one of fear, dread of the unknowns, sense of adventure, optimism about getting better, interest in who else is going to be there? Don't you think, too, about how your friends and family are going to respond to your hospital stay?

Going to the hospital in Boston and now again in New York taught me a lot about who I am. I learned quickly that, in many ways, I'm not much like other people. For example, it didn't occur to me to get into sleepwear or a robe or slippers at one o'clock in the afternoon. I don't like looking as if I'm sick when I feel fine, or staying in a place for four or five days without making it "mine" with some of my photos, my own soap, my bright-colored napkin and napkin ring from Elizabeth. I also don't like eating from a formica bed table without a tablecloth, or without some color around me. An operation doesn't make me feel "sick." I want to be in a nightgown only when I'm miserably sick and have to sleep all day. But, of course, I noticed I was the only dressed patient. Also I was the only patient, apparently, who brought along work. After all, I wasn't on a day off, and what would I do from 1:00 P.M. until Dan Rather at 7:00 if I didn't take my work? Sitting in the chair at the end of my bed, and using the bed table for my desk, I spread out the book I was working on and got right down to work. A doctor, clinical fellow, nurse, technician, or dietitian would rush in, look around, look at me, and with much impatience ask, "Where's the patient?"

"Right here. Me."

A disapproving eye would search me from head to toe, and I would quickly be ordered to get on the bed for questions or an examination. I did.

I was waiting for the anesthesiologist. I remember well that the worst part of going into surgery was trying to recover from the general anesthesia. I couldn't wake up after the operation in Boston. They kept calling my name, and I just couldn't come around. Even worse was the shot in my rear end before I left my room. So when the anesthesiologist came in before surgery, I explained I was a runner; the muscles back there must be hard because I ended up black and blue and sore for a week after they had had such an awful time getting the needle in my backside. Besides, I was calm before the operation and didn't want a sedative that hurts so much and gets me so tense.

"Okay, you don't have to have a sedative in your room."

"Okay?" That was easy.

"And furthermore, I'm only five feet and 110 pounds. I don't need as much anesthesia as normal-sized people. My body responds very quickly to any sedative, alcohol, a dentist's novocaine. It took me forever to recover the last time I had a general. Besides that I get very nauseous from anesthesia."

"You've got nothing to worry about! This is sweet stuff. You got anesthesia A the last time, and we give anesthesia B here at Sloan-Kettering. You'll see it's terrific. As long as you don't eat for twenty-four hours before the operation, you'll have no aftereffects."

My young South American roommate, Maria, was about a day ahead of me in surgery. She had been living in Hong Kong for the past few years, but her family was in Miami and New York and so gathered around her for this family tragedy. She was scared of everything, even of asking questions. I don't know Spanish, but I could make out her father's repetitive "Thank God, you're cured. . . . Thank God, you're cured." A warm person, he always nodded or said *buenos días* to me on his way to see his favorite daughter. I felt lucky to be sharing the same room with this cheerful, happy family.

There were lots of phone calls that night: from Bill, saying he'd be there after surgery; my mother and two of her Hardwick friends; and Lynne, my young filmmaker friend from ODN, the film production company where I had last worked, just before going to Paris.

I went to sleep feeling good.

Surgery was scheduled for around noon, so I got an early start on my work on the book I was writing, *College to Career*. When the technician and students and nurses and others came in to take some blood or my temperature or to ask questions, it was easy to get right back to my task. A little hunger was the only thing that made this morning different from other mornings. I was up and ready to get this cancer out of my body—now.

My third meeting with Dr. Sockol was the morning of surgery. Now we both knew he had the upper hand; our hellos and how-are-yous went very smoothly.

The stretcher guy, dressed in OR gear, came into my room with his stretcher on wheels. I was sitting in the chair at the end of my bed. He said, "You aren't supposed to be out of bed before surgery."

"I didn't have a sedative," I responded.

"You're supposed to. How can I take you to the OR? Get back in bed."

"I'll just get on the stretcher."

"You're supposed to get on the stretcher from the bed."

The technician did not like a patient getting on his stretcher from anywhere except that bed.

The waiting room outside the OR was cold. I mean cold!

"Do you want a blanket?" asked someone in white. "Please."

I'm in the operating room now, and it's cold here too. About five cheerful, very young people are talking to each other, teasing each other, asking about what they did last night. The lights are bright, straps all around me. I'm all goose pimples. They ask me all kinds of questions about Vermont, my children. Small talk, very lively, nothing-to-be-scared-of chitchat.

"Dr. Sockol will be here shortly," I'm told. In he comes. This time I'm as friendly as I get. He smiles and nods to the anesthesiologist, like a conductor starting his orchestra. . . . I'm wondering about all of the people around me. . . . I'm going fast . . . g-o-n-e.

No arguments with the stretcher man on my way out. No memory of anyone calling my name to awaken me. No memory of the changeover from stretcher to hospital bed in my own room. Betsy had come and gone. A nurse's voice said, "Don't worry. She's okay. She'll open her eyes soon."

The tweed sports coat sitting at the end of my bed said something. Just as I became aware that it was Bill's voice, and wanted to reach out for him, I needed to reach even more for something to throw up in. From nowhere came a little green plastic dish held in front of me at the same time I was lifted forward by a nurse. I heard Bill say, "Oh, the poor thing, she's going to be sick."

"Oh, Bill, I feel so miserable."

It must have been five or six o'clock, and I don't know when I focused, talked, and felt like drinking a little water, but it was certainly sometime before ten or eleven that night. What I do know is that I wanted my hand in Bill's: to take hold of that very familiar hand of his, a hand that had held mine for twenty-four years and knew better than anyone how to comfort me.

The very next morning a nurse's aide came in and announced that "we" were going to take a shower. A shower! I'm not even all here! I don't know how my arms and legs work; I haven't even washed my face yet! Somehow I was standing where she wanted me, with my drain tubes hanging outside and a drain flask hitched to me, and she was turning on the water. I trusted that I would get wet only what she had in mind to get wet. Reading my hesitancy and lack of enthusiasm for this collaborative task, she got a bright smile on her face and asked, "Where's that pretty French soap at?"

She got my attention. Wouldn't it be wonderful to feel and smell that smooth, sweet, luxurious Parisian soap on my skin? Wasn't she smart? And wasn't she thoughtful and creative to think of the very thing that would please me in this impossible shower?

My stomach recovered from acute nausea, and my hospital stay soon became more social than critical or hurtful. I knew from experience that I wouldn't have the results of the lab report to tell me the extent of my cancer for several more days. My room was filled with flowers, cards, and even balloons. A handful of balloon hearts with ribbon streamers were tied to my bed from Oralee, president of ODN, and her crew. ODN's Lynne Smilow had called the hospital to find out what time I had gone into surgery and what time I had come back to my room, and then reported to everyone in her company what was going on. I hadn't realized that so many friends had gone in with me.

After that memorable shower, I was expected to start right off with an exercise class, followed by a social worker's class, all required group work. It was interesting to get to know the other women and to see what the staff thought was important for us.

I put on my jeans, clogs, and a shirt and adjusted that drain flask under my shirt and went to class. A woman there asked how I got permission to be dressed. I responded that it didn't require permission. "I feel better in clothes, I'm not going to spend my money on a robe which I don't own, and I am concentrating on healing an incision that doesn't feel sick." The next day she, too, turned up in her clothes.

As soon as I began to feel better, I realized I had a major problem to start worrying about: to start role-playing the what-ifs, to start figuring out my plan A and plan B for handling my life if I have a "lymph node involvement," as they say in cancer talk. One of the main points I had learned the first time around is that breast cancer without lymph node involvement is a piece of cake, compared with breast cancer that has left the contained area and gone somewhere else (metastasized)—for example, progressed to the lymph nodes under the arm of the involved breast. Even if only one node is involved, it signifies travel. But if eight or ten or twelve are involved, the treatment usually continues after surgery.

Knowing that Dr. Sockol was out of town on Thursday, three days after surgery when the lab test results would be ready, I should have realized that Dr. Hellman was making more than a social call as I introduced him to Parker. Parker. Such an important friend since childhood, when his family had lived across the street from us in Hardwick. He went away to college when I was in the eighth grade, my very first college friend. It was from Parker that I first heard of and saw copies of the *New Yorker* and of *Theatre Arts*. And during all of those twenty-four Vermont years when I wanted to be in New York City, he would put me up in his apartment for the two nights and three workdays every month I spent in the city selling my book ideas or seeing my editors. He has always been in publishing, so he knew them all. He was more interested than anybody else in the world about how I sold my work. We'd have breakfast, and we'd talk and talk about whom I was going to see and, the next morning, about how it went. My life would be very different without Parker. When I was at my lowest during chemotherapy, a lunch with Parker always turned around my perspective and got me beyond myself—thinking of developing an idea and selling a book.

With Parker I never felt like a cancer victim, even with no hair and low energy. Dr. Hellman said he wanted to speak to me alone. Parker waited for me in the smoke-filled eighteenth-floor lounge. Dr. Hellman sat down in a chair at the end of the bed and motioned for me to sit beside him. Looking me straight in the eye, he said, "Your disease has progressed. You've got to have chemotherapy. All three levels of your lymph nodes are now involved." He put his hand on mine and added, "I'm sorry."

Questions came spilling out: "How can that be?" The first time you said I had all of the important conditions for getting rid of it forever. It was a tiny lump, the size of a BB. I had found it early. And it was treated right away. I'm not even supposed to have a recurrence! How can it have progressed so much? I thought attitude was important. I had the best attitude you can get: I was sure I'd never have it again. Where else can it be? Bones, other breast, lymph system, liver, lungs, brain. . . . Jesus! I don't believe in chemotherapy. I don't want all of those poisons in my body."

Dr. Hellman explained that I had a recurrence in spite of those three conditions because the particular cancer that I have has a component that almost always recurs. Regardless of treatment, whether radiation or surgery.

"Why didn't I know this before?"

With much empathy he explained, "Our research is new. We learned about this condition for recurrence three years after your treatment."

God! I tried to get Dr. Hellman to agree that the same component would still be present and that surgery or chemotherapy wouldn't do any good this time either. He wouldn't agree.

I walked in to the waiting room to get Parker, started back, my arm in his arm, and very quietly told him my devastating news. I didn't want to let go of his arm. I wanted his physical wellness and good health to flow through me through our interlocked arms. I wanted to hang on to his arm and keep walking around and around that floor. Slowly, talking in low voices, we continued our conversation as if it could have been about anything at all: a new movie, that new Off-Off Broadway play, my Prentice-Hall book. . . . Why, anyone looking at us would think we were just out for a stroll. And all the time we were figuring out what I could do to stop this progressing cancer that persists in threatening my life.

Friendships. Isn't it odd how so many friends can come together in this microscopic space—with two chairs and one tiny, narrow hospital bed?

Some friendships can get so deep. Parker's. Betsy's. Natalie's. Lyn's. And Marylynn's, as expressed through her letter and Saturday's visit. It's remarkable that communications can take place on this level. It's so satisfying, no matter what the issue. Other friends, though, seem to keep their distance. Still others want to be friends by glossing over and denying conflict. They just move right along, smiling away while such a hostile undercurrent is coming at me. I wonder why that is so offensive to me? Why do I always feel so compelled to confront it? Why can't I just let it go—sometimes? At least while I'm in the hospital fighting cancer.

Now I really have a problem. I've got to figure out what to do about progressing cancer. My life is going down right in front of my eyes, and I don't even feel it or look it—I'm the star in my exercise class!

François Truffaut died of cancer yesterday in Paris, fifty-two. I'm about fifty-two. Let's say I'll know more later, after I've seen the chemotherapist and had another meeting with Dr. Hellman about survival rates, prognosis, and my disease. Still, if I see my children's college graduation, an event that would be one of the highlights of my life; if I attend their weddings, see my children in love, and committed to that love; or if I ever see my children's children—then I will be very surprised.

What will not surprise me is excitement in daily living: the pure fun and enjoyment of being with friends and family. The pleasure that French language, bread, and wine and travel to France give me. Excitement with my work and with the work of RVer Annie, my cookbook company in Vermont. The strong, healthy feelings that come with jogging, tennis, skiing, walking, and exercise. And, of course, the community spirituality and inspiration of my church family. Small things too: greetings from complete strangers on the street, on the subway, at the hospital, in Central Park. Being thrilled by New York City's hustle: express subway, the very fastest ride from Grand Central to Fourteenth Street without stopping, making the light, running for the bus. Oh dear! All of that is plenty to live for.

I'm going home tomorrow. But I haven't even seen everybody who wanted to come to the hospital to see me. That's all there is to it? Well, all right. One last walk around the eighteenth floor with a Pennsylvania woman from my exercise class. She wants to talk about chemo. Her doctor didn't recommend it. She feels she should have it; after all, she has a lymph node involvement. We talk about the pros and cons. She thinks he didn't recommend it, because he thinks she's too old and can't "take it." This is exactly what I had read in an article in a breast cancer booklet published by the Chemotherapy Foundation and written by its president, Dr. Ezra M. Greenspan, oncologist and professor at Mount Sinai School of Medicine. He writes, "In women over fifty, a majority of oncologists avoid temporary side effects while sacrificing long-term survival. In other words, the better chance for cure is by-passed in many patients in favor of a more pleasant immediate lifestyle." He goes on to say, "Many patients are never clearly told of the actual pros and cons of treatment choices." Just like my new friend.

Even assuming that my eighteenth-floor mate may be right, I can't imagine anyone's wanting chemotherapy! Finally, I asked her, "What's your gut feeling, your intuition about it?" She responded very quickly, "I should have it." Then she gave a specific reason: "My grandson wouldn't be alive today if it wasn't for chemotherapy."

"And you want to be a good example for him, showing him grandma is getting chemo too?"

"Exactly."

"I'm going to tell my doctor tomorrow. I don't care how far I have to travel, and how hard it is. I am prepared to have chemotherapy—just like my grandson."

"Brava!"

Quitting Chemo

❖❀❖

"I quit."

"This is no way to live, even with cancer."

Two weeks after leaving the hospital, I had my first chemo hit, and one week later I said, "I'm resigning from this chemotherapy program. I refuse to stick my hand out again to take in poisonous chemicals that make me feel this sick!"

It was all decided. I consider myself a very healthy person, even though I had breast cancer five years ago. My first chemotherapy "hit" after surgery for recurrent breast cancer struck me with such force, packed such a wallop that until that moment I hadn't even known it was possible to be that wiped out. Radiation and surgery were a piece of cake compared with chemo. After all, I was the star in my postsurgical exercise class. I'm a runner. A tennis player. A woman in good shape. A woman who watches her weight and health and who has always been physically fit. How could some so-called treatment come along and knock me off my feet, paying no attention whatever to my physical fitness?

I wanted out. Those killer drugs had nothing to do with me. It took only one hit for me to find out that chemo is as tough as cancer. I wanted to be back in Vermont, recuperating from surgery and as far away from chemotherapy as I could get. As my friend Natalie wrote me, "I know you wish someone could give you a hug and kiss and make it all go away." Oh yes—that's exactly what I wished. I wrote my letter of resignation to the chemotherapist and took off for Vermont as fast as People Express could take me. This is what I had on my mind—and in my gut:

November 15, 1984

Dear Dr. Minelli:

It is with mixed feelings that I send you my resignation from your experimental chemotherapy program.

I cannot accept your mind-set of a totally scientific chemical model of treatment, because it is the very antithesis of what feels right for my body and soul. Therefore, I regret that I am unable to finish something that I began.

I am going to turn to an environmental, nurturing, physical-fitness model, the only treatment to which I can commit my life. I want to build up (not completely destroy through drugs) my natural immunity system, even as I am aware that Dr. Hellman pointed out to me that, until now, my immunity system hasn't been working that well for me.

I went into my first chemo encounter (November 8), with a positive and curious attitude. The administration by the head nurse was instructive and went very smoothly. I left at about 6:30 P.M., still curious and expecting to tolerate the dosage. About five hours later I was completely wiped out by throwing up on the hour for twenty-four hours (in spite of the prescribed medicine, which I took every four hours), followed by twenty-four hours of nausea in general, unable to drink even a sip of water to flush out the drugs as quickly as possible (to prevent damage to my liver and kidneys, as you had suggested). By the third day I was sick from the sheer lack of food! Now it's the seventh day, and my sense of smell and taste are sickening to live with. This reaction is from a runner who recovered from surgery faster than anyone around.

As I lay in bed, trying to imagine the poisons raging through my body killing off the cancer cells, all I could think of was you sitting there saying to me, "I wish I could tell you that this treatment will help, but for the majority of people it doesn't." And my response, "Well, what about my specific case? What about helping me, a fifth-year radiated recurrent breast cancer case?" And your reply, "We have even less data for radiated people, five years out."

My gut response is that chemotherapy does not make sense for me. Chemicals have nothing to do with the direction I want to go for reducing my possible cancer cells.

I am eager to start exercising again (I started yesterday).

I am eager to take my vitamins (I was told not to during chemo). I am eager to think of my body as capable of fighting off whatever it has to in order for me to live a life where I can stand the smells and tastes.

I am a writer. My current work includes a cookbook. Writing about food with a bandana around my nose

because I cannot stand the smell of air or the thought of
cooking is not my idea of a quality life. Yours sincerely,
                                    Joyce Slayton Mitchell
                                    c.c.: Samuel Hellman, M.D.

I talked to Bill about it. A professor at the University of
Vermont, he still lives on the farm where we raised our two
children. Three weeks after surgery and ten days after my
first chemo hit, I desperately needed to touch home base.
Bill cautioned me to wait until I felt better before making any
decision about giving up on chemotherapy. I waited. It took
ten days to recover from that first chemo wipeout. Bill was
going to be away for a few days and asked if I'd come home
to feed Wewak, our dog, named for the nearest port in New
Guinea, where we had spent two years of our lives in the
bush on an anthropological expedition.

Yeah, I could do that. I wanted to be in Vermont feeding
Wewak. To touch the land I know by heart. To walk my
woods. Smell my meadows and pastures and dirt road. Talk
to Tressa Grant, my neighbor, and walk by her henhouse.
Feel winter coming on. Listen to the brook by the falls and
water hole where our children used to swim. Work on RVer
Annie & Company, the cookbook-publishing business I had
started just before my cancer was discovered. See my
mother. See my aunts and uncles, my cousins, and great-
aunt, and my mother's neighbors in Hardwick, where I grew
up—seven miles from the farm where I raised my children.

Getting in touch with where you come from is not the
same as wanting to live there. It's more like college students
coming home for the first time. They want to make sure their
homes are as they remembered them, knowing all the while,
though, they would suffocate if they stayed. Their first time
home often frees them to get on with their new life at college.
Can you think of the place that feels best to you in a crisis?

Is it your current home? Your living room? Your bedroom? Is it a relative's home, or one in a town where you used to live? Is it the house where you grew up? Or your first home? As much as I wanted to leave the isolation of our Vermont farm, and as much as I loved my new, fast-paced life in New York City, I wanted to be on that farm right then.

I don't think I'll ever forget the warm bubble-bath water that covered my incision for my first bath since surgery. The bathtub stands next to double windows on its clawed feet, in a room bigger than my Manhattan bedroom, on the second floor of Bill's hundred-year-old farmhouse. The bathroom windows overlook a high meadow, a couple of wild apple trees, and a stand of spruces on the hilly horizon. I slid down into the tub. Watching my incision going under the rising water over my chest, I scooped some of the bubbles to cover it, took a deep breath and r-e-l-a-x-e-d. . . . Ahhhhhhhhhhhh deep, deep, down into my very center—for the first time since learning that I had cancer. Again.

That first evening in Vermont I built a wood fire in the stove where I had burned eight cords of wood during my last winter in Vermont (non-wood-burning readers of this book should know that one cord equals a pile of wood measuring four by four by eight feet). I thought of the cold winter nights when I was awakened by the sound of the oil furnace going on. Bounding out of bed, I raced to stoke the fire so that I wouldn't have to pay for oil, accepting my own challenge to heat the house solely with wood. God! New York City is different!

My aunt Eunice brought dinner—everything from Cabot cheese and filet mignon with a béarnaise sauce to a great big sweet dessert, because I had told her I craved sweets since that first chemo hit.

That big sweet dessert was a chocolate cream pie, with perfect Crisco crust and real whipped cream. We sat around the table in the kitchen. My cousin, too, and Hazel, Hardwick's artist. Her paintings surround me in my six-by seven-foot city bedroom. A huge bouquet of zinnias beside me; a smaller version of the same flowers in front of me; the Walden church above that; Hardwick's Main Street above my filing cabinet on the other side; Hardwick Academy, where everyone of us in the kitchen had gone to school, now torn down; and Hazel's self-portrait. A primitive profile with one eye looking straight out at me! Every time I sold a book, I bought one of Hazel's paintings. But I had never been so enclosed by them or enjoyed them so much before my move to New York's tiny spaces.

At the kitchen table, my Vermont family and friends wanted to hear all about chemotherapy. I gave them my resignation letter to read. They took their clues from me and decided I was right. They wouldn't choose chemotherapy either. It was the unhealthiest thing they'd ever heard of too.

The weekend was permeated by my questions: Had I made the right decision? Or was I just acting out? Was I looking for control in a situation where there is none? Would cancer symptoms appear if I didn't take it? If I did? Would I live as long if I didn't take chemo? Would the chemo make enough of a difference to be worthwhile? Walking the familiar logging trails in my woods helped me grapple with these questions. And working on my cookbook business with my neighbor Beulah Ryder, who served me applesauce with saltines for dessert, made me feel stronger and healthier again. Being in Vermont felt good. Felt right. The highlight of my weekend was "The Tea."

Phyllis Zechinelli, Hardwick's English war bride, had asked my mother if I wanted a tea when I was home. Yes! I wanted to see the women in the village where I had grown up, my schoolteachers, the women who had phoned me at Sloan-Kettering and sent me cards and notes when I was dealing with surgery, this time for a modified radical mastectomy.

I sat in the rocker. Squarely opposite me, seated three across the sofa were Mrs. Bemis, Mrs. Holcomb, and Mrs. Allbee, my mother's friends who had known me since I was born. Eve Bemis and her husband ran the local five-and-ten store in Hardwick when I was growing up. I can remember buying my mother a blue bottle of Evening in Paris from Eva's store when I was about seven. Fran Holcomb and her husband ran Hardwick's undertaking business, and she also played the church organ. Esther Allbee came to Hardwick in the 1920s with her parents, who ran the Hardwick Inn, and she was Parker's fourth-grade teacher. These were the women who lived on my street and who had cheered me on at all of my high school basketball games; knew I had caught the biggest fish in town the first day of trout fishing when I was eight; watched me leave Vermont at seventeen to go away to Ohio, where no one had gone before; waved good-bye when I was the first person in Hardwick to go to Europe "who didn't have to"; bought the Cloverine salve, garden seeds, and Christmas cards I sold according to the season to earn money to go away to summer camp.

Also at the tea was Mrs. Cobb, my English, Latin, and French teacher. I grew up with her children, sharing paper routes, books, skiing, and sex information and waiting during the war for vanilla ice cream to come to Hardwick once a week—on Saturdays. There, too, was Mrs. Mosher, my seventh-grade English teacher, whose eighth-grade son was the first true love of my life. I promised myself I would always remember when I grew up how it felt to be in love, and it definitely was not puppy love, as my mother claimed.

In their eighties, these women talked of travel and their Florida plans for the winter. "I'm going to stay right here in Hardwick," said Eva. "I'm sick of Florida. Sally, if you'd stay we could keep our bridge club going all winter." My mother replied, "Well, I'm going to Florida one more year, and you girls know that there's not one of us who can remember a card in our hand." In her nineties, Mrs. Cobb told me that she was Governor Kunin's oldest volunteer and asked if I'd heard that she was going to the governor's ball to celebrate her victory.

Phyllis's table was elegant, set with a silver tea service, linens, and fine china. But first we had sherry in the living room, followed by a buffet of cucumber and salmon open tea sandwiches, and nut bread with cream cheese. There was lots of talk and then the pièce de résistance, an authentic British trifle, served with more tea. We discussed Madeleine Kunin, Vermont's first woman governor, but spoke very little about cancer or sickness and not at all about chemotherapy. I sat there without drinking the sherry, not yet used to being in a social situation without drinking and thought what it would be like to go six months without it. I wished I could have a good belt of that sherry or, better yet, a nice cold beer from Phyllis's refrigerator. Soon, though, I forgot the booze. I just loved being there. I sat back and relaxed, listening and watching.

As they left, all said how good I looked and used words like *bravery, courage,* and *hope;* otherwise, though, cancer and its ugly recurrence were left unsaid.

On Sunday I went to church, feeling immersed in the familiar and safe, a little like my bathtub in a funny way. That night I was back on the plane heading for New York City. I had made the right decision—*this* was the way to live. Even if it would turn out to mean a shorter life.

Confident that this was the right choice for me, I got back to New York to find a letter from Dr. Hellman. This is what he said:

November 18, 1984

Dear Joyce,
    I am sorry to hear about your unfortunate experiences with chemotherapy, but I am writing to urge you to

continue your treatment. While I can understand your feelings, some of the statements are not accurate and may lead you to an erroneous conclusion. First, you indicate that this is an experimental program; it is not. While physical fitness is important, I must emphasize to you that, despite your body's immune system, this tumor has recurred and progressed. Clearly, the immune system is not sufficient. Exercise and normal nutrients are fine. I believe Dr. Minelli can make some modifications in the chemotherapy to reduce the side effects to some extent. Unfortunately, these cannot be obviated completely, but I believe the net gain is worth the discomfort. I wish you were right in assuming that the "environmental, nurturing, physical-fitness model" would work, but I worry that in doing so you will deny a treatment that has evidence to support it and that I believe is not directly competitive.

I hope you will reconsider your decision. In any case, please keep in touch. Personal regards.

Sincerely yours,
Sam

Thanksgiving Time: The Big Decision

◇❀◇

The best Thanksgiving I ever remember at the farm was the year when Bill and I took the children to my cousin's farm in Cabot to pick out our turkey. Alive, I mean. We looked them all over out there in the turkey yard and found the slowest-moving, fattest one, which we thought would feed twenty-two people. That was the year I got a piece of venison from Harold Nunn, our TV antenna repairer, whom I had grown up with in Hardwick. I wanted to make venison mincemeat pies. And the Irishes were coming from New York City. That meant that I could make something special with our lamb hearts and kidneys for a first course, because I knew that it takes a New Yorker to love innards. We raised sheep and ate about seven of them a year. I remember that Thanksgiving as another one when we couldn't have dinner until six, because my dad hadn't shot his deer yet, and on this the last day of deer season he wouldn't come in until dark, at four o'clock. And that was the year we took the picture of Elizabeth Dix with her forebears: George Dix, her grandfather; Laura Dix, her great-grandmother; Rachael Dix, her great-great aunt; and Thurman Dix, her great-great uncle.

I can just smell that Thanksgiving kitchen with everything cooking at once, steaming up the windows. And I can see winter coming on in the kitchen, where I spent most of my time with the children: Ned reading in his favorite corner of the kitchen sofa, bookshelves under the window, where the frost crept indoors and iced the electrical outlets, and on the floral-papered walls the warm-looking oils of Bessie Drennan, Vermont's Grandma Moses.

Thanksgiving always brought the excitement of deer season, of the first snow that would "stay," sometimes of the first skiing of the season, and always of the wonderful change of the New Yorkers coming up to Vermont with all those marvelous breads and wines and stories of movies, restaurants, jobs, people, and plays with them. We never had a Thanksgiving without Diane and Loomis Irish and their two children, Mark and Carol, just a few years older than ours. It was from Diane that I learned what children read and wear in New York, what lessons they take, what they do at their parties, and what happens in private education. We never had a Christmas without the Irishes, either, but that was always at their Vermont farm, with a tree bigger than the room they had it in.

So the first year I was in New York, 1983, happened to be the first time that the Irishes, Joyce, Ned, and Elizabeth weren't in Vermont for Thanksgiving. Luckily for me, I got to be with the Irishes and with Elizabeth. We went out to Tuxedo Park, about an hour out of the city, with an old-world look of lake and mountain and walks. Such beauty in the familiar family: being with our children, who had left home, meeting their college friends and listening to their latest adventures.

The worst Thanksgiving I ever remember was the second Thanksgiving away from Vermont in 1984. I went to the Irishes' again, this time by myself, since Elizabeth and Ned were both in California. I had a lot on my mind because I had to decide what to do about Sam Hellman's letter received a week before. I felt very heavy, as if the decision I was about to make was the only real one in my life. Everything in me was so against chemotherapy, yet everything in me was so for Dr. Samuel Hellman. I knew he was a man I trusted and admired, and yet I hated what he prescribed.

Once I was at home with the Irishes, Diane suggested we take a brisk walk to see the lovely trees and lake and to feel the peace of the bucolic park. She always has a lot to think about, being head of the lower school at Chapin, a private school for girls in New York City. I love hearing her stories and problems and solutions, and watching her enthusiasm for children and education. Over the years I've heard such detail that I feel I could go into her school and know where everything and who everybody is.

When we got to the boat house, we sat in the sun for a few minutes and I read Diane my letter to Dr. Minelli, my chemotherapist, and my letter from Dr. Hellman. I knew what her response would be: she just couldn't imagine my having a choice!

Diane was aghast the minute I told her that I wasn't going to buy a wig, that if this is what chemotherapy did to a person, the world ought to know—people ought to be able to look at the baldness caused by such a dramatic and deadly drug! She just couldn't understand my logic. I said I'd wear bandanas and hats, so why spend $50 on a wig I'd never need again? Oh, the terrible thought of that false hair on my head, not to mention how it would look! Everyone would know I have cancer, so why not the bald head or a hat? Diane explained to me that I could probably get a wig for $25, that the convenience of not having to figure out what I'd put on my head each time would be worth it to me. She convinced me.

That night was the loneliest night of my life. For the first time I cried with fear. I thought one way and then the other. The room was cold and the outdoors black. The wind in the trees was icy and alienating inside and out. And it was so very, very dark. I was of two minds. I felt I was going to die if I didn't have chemotherapy. On the other hand I was pretty sure I would die from the chemotherapy. Part of my fear was about being in that bed alone. People always say that in the face of major decisions you're always alone even if you're with someone. But I wasn't even with someone. It was just me. It was the night before Thanksgiving, the first time I had ever been without my family at a holiday. Thanksgiving was such a big event in my family. I thought back to when I was little and went to my grandmother's house in Hardwick, then to when I was married and had my grandmother at my house all of those years. Now Bill was at the farm and probably serving pasta for Thanksgiving. Ned and Elizabeth were in Santa Cruz and very likely were not even celebrating. As for me, I was with the Irishes, which was certainly the next-best thing to being with family. Still, none of us were in Vermont, where we belonged for Thanksgiving and Christmas. Oh God! Is this how lonely people feel all the time? I woke up before dawn, reached for my pencil and paper, and began to write:

Tuxedo Park
Thanksgiving Day

Dr. Samuel Hellman
Dear Sam,
    I'll keep my next chemo appointment.
    Thank you for your thoughtful letter.
    I understand that I can't "know" all I want to know to

make good decisions about my treatment. I understand that I've asked all the questions I can think of, and still have no sense of where I am with my condition. I understand that I won't be able to feel "on top" (in control) through more information.

I trust you. I know that, given the unknowns, you will make the best decision available. I believe that there is no one in the world with more information, better judgment, or more interest and concern for my health than you. Your laugh, humor, and life sparkle add a dimension of warmth that make you an outstanding physician.

Then why am I in such a dilemma? Because chemotherapy feels so unhealthy. It doesn't make sense to me. I'm afraid that it's going to kill me—wiping out my good cells, even when nobody knows (a) whether I have microscopic cancer cells and (b) whether they are going to progress to symptoms. I hate the sickness that chemo brings to me. I hate looking at my calendar filled with hospital and doctor appointments—a medical focus in my life. I hate that the majority of people are not helped by chemo. I don't want six months of chemo (a sickly life) if I'm in that majority that chemo doesn't help. Worse, I don't want chemo to kill me.

I like the way you think. You don't think with an either-or mentality, as I have. In the course of the next treatment, I'll try harder to bring more of my sense of good health to it with exercise, vitamins, and a healthful diet.

I so hope that I will be able to bring together your concern that I get all the medical treatments available to me with my concern that I get a "healthy" environment that makes sense to me.

Happy Thanksgiving, Sam.

Yours sincerely,
Joyce

Okay. That's it. I'll go with him, for better or for worse. Nothing to do with chances, or options, or odds, or truth. All to do with trust. And I'll make this decision for all my cancer treatments. I can't go through this agony with each chemo hit, or the agony will be my death!

Relax. . . . Just a little.

Look, the sky is clearing; those evergreen treetops from my window have just been struck by the rising sun. There's a true Thanksgiving sky. One more letter. I'll tell my aunt Eunice what I've decided.

Dear Aunt Eunice,

I'm trying to work out my chemo treatment decision and figure out where I can make changes that will enable me to fight the strongest-possible battle against cancer.

One problem I see from Dr. Hellman's letter to me is that I have been polarizing my options—chemo versus healthy. He was astute and turned that thought around to say that he didn't see my views as competitive.

In other words, I should do it all. Chemo plus exercise plus vitamins plus healthy diet. I've just decided that I can give it another try. I'm proud of myself for being open to his letter, for not taking the rigid stance that I've made up my mind and already said no. Even more important, I'm not enjoying the role of saying no to the top cancer institute more than I'd enjoy the role of fighting cancer in a traditional way.

I felt so alone last night and early this morning, as I worked out this chemotherapy problem—even with so many loving friends and relatives in my life. Interesting how personal and alone this tough "working out" is. There just isn't someone else who can help, who can be responsible, who can take the consequences of this and other critical decisions in life. My aloneness in the universe is so clear to me on this Thanksgiving Day. And

*yet, I don't feel isolated or abandoned by friends! I know
I can count on you and Bill and my children and mother
and on my brother and aunts and cousins and Diane and
Loomis and Lyn and Parker to back me—whatever way I
go. I'm confident about the love and caring of my family
and friends.*

*I've been in the depths of despair, as the psalmists
would say. I don't feel that way now. I like my decision.
I'm proud of having expanded my view even in a crunch.
I'm looking forward to a run (first since surgery) and to a
walk with Diane in this beautiful Tuxedo Park, on this
clear, sunny day. I'm looking out the window of a home
designed for and lived in by Emily Post. Which reminds
me of manners. And your home ec classes.*

*Thanks for being so with me this Thanksgiving
morning.*

Love and thoughts,
Joyce

I'll read until everyone gets up. Take another walk with
Diane. Tell her what I've decided.

The Second Hit

◇✿◇

Thorazine?? Isn't that what they give psychotic patients? Isn't that what state hospitals give out for schizophrenia (not that I know what schizophrenics are)? Remember *One Flew Over the Cuckoo's Nest?* Isn't that what Jack Nicholson's doctor prescribed to keep him in line? God! I don't want Thorazine!

Sitting in Dr. Minelli's office with my list of questions written in my beautiful Paris notebook, I told him about my reaction from the first hit. The chemical takeover lasted twenty-four hours, hours of active vomiting, followed by two days of no food and a third day of total weakness.

That's when I noticed his expensive shoes. I just couldn't take my eyes off those cordovan wing tips, more like a million-dollar-club insurance salesman's than a doctor's, especially such a young doctor's. I'd surveyed other Sloan-Kettering doctors' shoes, and I'd seen a lot of laid-back L. L. Bean moccasin- or topsider-types on the younger men; plain cordovans or Gucci loafers on a few of the grown-up preppies; and even scuffy cordovans for an academic look. I had even seen a pair or two of black dress shoes on the surgeons. But wing tips?

The expensive look was not what attracted me to his wing tips. It was the position he kept them in during our conference that stole my concentration. Dr. Minelli always sat on the edge of his chair facing me, with his feet visible from the front of his desk way around the corner and pointing toward the door. It was if he were on a racing block, ready to run as soon as I got my last question out, signaling GO! It was the body language of a man who definitely had better things to do than explain the drugs and the management of their side effects to one patient. As I was trying to pretend I didn't notice his expensive shoes poised to run out the door, he first suggested Thorazine.

Dr. Minelli told me that if I was that nauseous after taking his prescribed Compazine, it was obvious that the Compazine was not an effective antinausea drug for me, so I was to get a shot of Thorazine and to pick up a prescription of Reglan in the hospital pharmacy, to take in pill form when I got home.

I had so many questions to ask him that I thought telling him that I didn't want Thorazine would push him over his tolerance level, so I let it go. If you're a chemo patient and have a great variety of anticancer drugs and another variety of drugs to inhibit side effects, you'll probably agree how hard it is to try to figure out which drug questions are most important for you to ask in the limited time you know you'll have your doctor's attention:—that brief moment before he runs out the door. After all, what did I know about Thorazine except for my impression from Jack Nicholson and hearsay? Besides, I'd just written him a letter that I was sure would put me on his top ten list of most difficult patients.

November 24, 1984

Dear Dr. Minelli:

I have decided to give it another try, as scheduled on Thursday, November 29, at 3:30.

I asked you about relaxing techniques when I first met you, and you told me that arrangements can be made for me to learn about them at Memorial. I arrived at the chemotherapy unit to take my first chemo treatment without hearing any more about this technique. When I asked a nurse if it wasn't too late to be finding out about ways to relax to reduce the side effects, she said they had a special nurse for this process but didn't say how I was to contact the nurse. When I was actually having the drugs administered, I asked again and learned that one nurse, who happens to be on vacation now, handles that.

I don't consider the above a "program" at Sloan-Kettering for helping with side effects if (a) I've asked about it four times and received no information about how to get it, (b) it's dependent upon one nurse, who may or may not be there and available, and (c) there are no provisions for all chemotherapy patients to learn about it–no phone number, person, or simple handout sheet.

In other words, if there's no access to the program, I consider it to be nonexistent. Given all the patients who may not have read about relaxing techniques for the reduction of side effects, those who wouldn't dream of asking "the doctor" for what wasn't offered, and those who would never ask a second time, I think it's a shocking statement to have to make about Memorial Sloan-Kettering, the most prestigious cancer center in the world.

*I am taking the time and energy to write to you about
this situation in hopes that you may initiate a change.
Not for me alone, but for me and all the chemotherapy
patients who could be benefiting by stress reduction
during their long, hard battle with chemotherapy.*

*I think that the least that could be offered is a
one-page handout telling about relaxation and whatever
else you do, to be given to the patient before she or he
gets to the unit for the drugs.*

*Sincerely,
Joyce Slayton Mitchell*

Well, even with this letter, I still didn't want to be on Dr.
Minelli's list of ten most difficult patients. After all, I wanted
to get along with this man who was prescribing me all that
poison!

Here are my questions and his answers. Actually, I didn't
get all of these answers at once. As you will know from your
experience in asking questions, the best way to get the information you want is to ask no more than five questions at a
time, no matter what kind of doctor you have. Even though
professionals in the health world tell you to be sure and ask
questions, they really don't mean it. When you get to the fifth
question in a single encounter, you begin to feel a strong
pressure to let the busy doctors get on with their important
work.

In a series of, say, three or four meetings with my chemotherapist when the drugs were prescribed, two or three
phone calls, and a letter or two, here's what I found out
about chemotherapy:

"Dr. Minelli, can you tell if the chemotherapy is working
as we go along?"

"Not really. The only way we can tell is through a negative

response, when a cancer symptom appears in spite of the chemotherapy. And then, of course, we don't proceed with the chemotherapy."

"You mean if I get a lump in my other breast, we'd know that chemo wasn't working?"

"Exactly."

"How do you know which drugs to give me? Do you change them along the way?"

"The choice of anticancer drugs for each patient depends on the type and location of the cancer, its state of development, how it affects normal body functions, and the general health of the patient. You may be treated with one drug or a combination of drugs. Yes, I'll change the dosage of the drugs you get from a very strong one in the first phase, given to you in three-week intervals, to a lower one, given to you on a weekly basis in phase two. The second phase is marked by more frequent treatments but will be much easier on your system."

"Will I gain weight or get bloated from these drugs?"

"Not necessarily. Individuals vary on weight gain and loss. However, some drugs often increase appetite, Prednisone, for example."

"What happens after six months of chemo, when my program is finished?"

"Most physicians have a follow-up procedure and like to see their patients every three to six months, depending on the case. At that time there are blood tests, scans, mammograms, and X rays, which we use to detect the symptoms. Otherwise, once the chemo is over, we wait and watch for the symptoms."

"Why is my white blood count down? Why doesn't my immune system produce more white blood cells?"

"Because all three of your drugs—Adriamycin, Cytoxan, and 5-FU—lower your blood count. That's one of their side effects."

"How many white blood cells do I have? How many are the finger prickers looking for?"

"Well, the average range of white blood cells is from 4,500 to 11,000. We usually look for a count of at least 3,000. The nurses and technicians refer to the blood count as "3.6" or "4" and drop the thousand. Therefore, they would tell you if you were under 3, there would be no chemo until your count was above 3.

"What does it mean to me if it goes below 3? Why can't I have chemo anyway? What can I do to get my blood count back up to where it should be?"

"Joyce, the danger is general infection. When your white blood count is down, your immune system can't fight off common colds, ordinary germs that cause infections from a scratch or a burn. It isn't safe to be in the everyday germ world without the protection of your white blood cells. In general, there is nothing you can do to hasten the buildup of your white blood cells, but I agree with you that eating well probably helps. However, there is no research to show that any particular diet will increase the white blood count."

"Will my stomach always be affected by these chemo drugs? Will I vomit for hours and hours each time?"

"Probably, since you responded so violently, but many people have very little or no nausea. The cause of your nausea is that Adriamycin is a very strong drug acting against the fast-growing cancer cells, but it affects all fast-growing cells, not just the cancer cells. Other fast-growing cells in your body are the lining of your stomach and the hair-growing cells."

"Dr. Minelli, Can I leave the program for a week in February? Does the exact three-week interval make a difference? What about when the blood count is down and I have to skip a week because of that?"

"I've heard many chemotherapists offer varying opinions on this, but, yes, you can take a week off in February. I don't think we know enough about chemotherapy to know if the precise time makes a lot of difference. I'd like to get the first three hits within the first three months, but I'm not particular about the day."

"How about taking chemo on a trip with me? Can I take the chemo with me if I go to Australia for a month? Can I go a month without chemo?"

"Now you're pushing it, Joyce. No, you can't go a month without it in the first phase. We'll wait and see how you respond before we make any decisions about the second phase, when you'll be on a weekly program."

"In what ways does stress affect outcome of chemo? I read a lot about using relaxing techniques so that the chemo side effects are not so bad. Do some of your patients practice a relaxation program? Does it make a difference in their side effects?

"Yes, we have a nurse at Sloan-Kettering who trains patients in relaxation. If you want to see her before the next therapy, I'll get her name for you. We don't know if it makes a difference in side effects. There's just no hard data to support it."

"I don't think of chemotherapy as something that's helping me; I think of it as something that's doing me in. Do you find a lot of patients who misplace their hate against cancer with this procedure?"

"Sure they do."

"Dr. Minelli, will my response to chemo be easier on me now than last time? Will my body get used to these poisons? Can I expect to work on a regular basis during chemo?"

"People vary, as I've said. But most of my patients work all the time. They get their therapy just before the weekend and go back to work on Monday. I have many in high-pressured jobs who don't miss any work."

"Speaking of working, how do exercise, jogging, tennis, and skiing affect chemo patients?"

"Whatever feels right for you is what you should try. Many patients exercise, although most don't jog or feel like doing vigorous exercise in the first phase of the program. Using your body can promote self-esteem, help you get rid of tension and anger. Exercise builds your appetite and helps you sleep soundly."

"I've read a few controversial articles about vitamin C. Since I tend to be a vitamin nut, I'd like to know how vitamins, especially C, affect my chemo program."

"I get a lot of questions about vitamin C. This is the point: we know that Cytoxan or any other drug reacts a certain way in your body against cancer cells. We do not know how it reacts when mixed with vitamins. I'd prefer that you not take vitamins; they could negate your chemotherapy."

"Good Lord! I certainly don't want to negate all of these horrendous treatments! How about coming here and getting home alone? Can I come alone? Will the reaction time always be the same? Will I have time to get home before the reaction?"

"I think it's best if someone comes with you during the first phase, until you see how you respond to the chemicals. When you get on the second phase, which will be much easier on your system, you can probably come alone."

"Alcohol. Dr. Minelli, tell me about alcohol."

"Don't drink while on chemotherapy. Doctors vary on this, but the point is that the liver responds to alcohol before it responds to any other drug. If you drink, your liver can't get rid of the chemo drugs, and they sit in the tissues of your kidneys, bladder, and liver and can be very harmful. You need as strong a liver as possible to process the chemo drugs. A little bit of alcohol damages the liver a little bit. A little more damages the liver a little more. When you're on some drugs such as Methotrexate and Prednisone or Methotrexate and Purinethol, it's important not to drink any alcohol, including wine and beer."

"You mean I can't just put a little wine in my water at dinner?"

"It would ruin the wine!"

"But it sure improves the water!"

It turned out that this discussion of alcohol was purely a theoretical exercise. If there was anything I couldn't tolerate while on chemo, it was alcohol in any form.

Soon after I collected this information from Dr. Minelli, the *New York Times* reported an interview with Dr. James F. Holland, chemotherapist from Mount Sinai Medical Center, in New York City. He is known for thinking that most chemo should be harder and stronger! He tells his patients, "The thing to remember is that the deadliest thing about cancer chemotherapy is not the chemo. The deadliest thing is the cancer." I try to remember that. He went on to say, "If chemotherapists cause short-term harm, it is for the long-term benefit." I try to remember that, too. What I try to remember most of all, and I bet you do, too, if you're a chemo patient, is that "the quality of your life is important to you, but so is a long life."

Bill called from Vermont to say he was coming to New York City and wanted to come to my second chemo hit with me. He planned to meet me at Sloan-Kettering, and knowing how curious he is about how everything works, I thought it would be interesting to hear his observations of the process. It helps to stand back and get perspective with an anthropologist around. Besides that, regardless of our divorce, it would feel good to have Bill with me.

In all the commotion and excitement and things to do just before getting chemo—the finger stick, weight, blood pressure, time with Dr. Minelli—I forgot that Bill is always late. When we were married, it always drove me crazy. Being divorced helps in our different expectations of each other. When he wasn't there after I qualified for the second round,

I went to the chemo unit. Connie called me into the inner sanctum, and I was ushered to one of those long-term, big lounge chairs to get started. Just as the nurse was finding the biggest and best vein on the back of my hand, Bill hurried in. He had been lost in the other building. He looked fresh and scrubbed, as he always does, and so academic in his tweeds and scarf and with his very animated face. The nurse was impressed that I had such a good-looking man with me, I could tell. She stuck the needle in the best-looking vein she could find, taped it down, gave it a test run with water, put in the real thing, and rushed off to be with another patient. I noticed the vein swelling and called out to her to come look. She said the needle had "blown" the vein, and she quickly removed it. I just hate all of that!

I was in a sweat and said to Bill, "everyone thinks that cancer is the horror story, but it's these little things that aren't anywhere near life-threatening that drive you crazy. Like having to find another vein and to stick the back of your hand twice. Wouldn't you think that just treating cancer would overshadow a little thing like that? It doesn't!"

We had a good laugh. He was impressed that I had noticed so quickly that the needle wasn't working.

After the drip started working properly, the first drug, Cytoxan, opened my nasal and sinus passages, letting the whole world of smells and cold metallic shudders into my system. It wasn't nearly as fascinating as the first time. This time the red syringe of Adriamycin, the drug that produces total hair loss, looked like red for danger. After things got settled down with the easy 5-FU for the long drip, the pharmacist happened to walk by, so I asked him to tell me about Reglan. Was it a lot better than Compazine for fighting nausea?

He replied, "Reglan? You can't be taking Reglan, because I've just drawn up a shot of Thorazine for you, and they don't mix."

"What do you mean they don't mix?"

"It's too complicated for your CNS."

"What's my CNS?"

"Central nervous system."

"Jesus!" I couldn't believe it and didn't know what to do.

"If you're sensitive to medication, the Thorazine will put you to sleep before you get home."

God! Just what I thought. I didn't want it in the first place!

And then the nurse chimed in with her two cents: "Reglan will give you the jitters." All of this talk certainly got my mind off cancer. I figured I'd be admitted to the nearest state hospital and die there of a mix-up in my CNS before I had time to throw up the chemicals.

All of this pharmaceutical conversation occurred about 6 P.M., after Dr. Minelli had gone home. So I scrapped the Thorazine, and as soon as Bill and I got home, I took two little Reglans, not wanting to take so much I'd have the jitters to keep me awake all night long with the vomiting. While I was getting the last of the drips, another patient, a friendly young woman in her early thirties, leaned toward me and said, "You're having trouble with nausea? I'll tell you the secret. Bread sticks. Here, have one before they take the drip out. I brought some extras. I start eating bread sticks the last five minutes of the drip and eat several more, along with plenty of water to flush out the chemicals, and I don't have any trouble at all. Here, take another one; you'll need several to work."

Eleven P.M. Ohhhhh, gross—bread sticks. I'll taste them forever. Don't say the word. Without taking any more antinausea medication, I continued throwing up every hour on the hour for the next twenty-four. All the same, I wasn't as sick as the first time. I felt stronger and didn't mind it quite as much. I think the first time the Compazine had made me sick in between the bouts of vomiting and added to the weakness without taking away any of the nausea.

Knowing what was going to happen helped. I wasn't as scared that the nausea would go on forever, although every day something new happened. If you're a chemo patient, you'll remember with me the heightened smells that were sickening, the mouth sores, the sore scalp, or the general fatigue. I decided that when I went in to Dr. Minelli next time, I'd put the Raglan on his desk and ask him, "Just when did you plan for me to take this seventeen dollars' worth of medicine? If I had taken the shot you prescribed, I would have been asleep before I could have opened the bottle. I think your whole concern is with the main event, the chemo, and you just doesn't give a damn about side effects." Besides that, the nurse had said to me, "Listen, with the amount of drugs they're giving you, there isn't any medication you can take to ease nausea." I thought she was probably right. And if so, I'd rather just go without.

By Saturday, I was thinking of my oatmeal, and on Sunday I added apples and oranges—recovery. Just in time for Parker's Christmas party!

The Help Center

❖❀❖

Quick Reference

QUESTIONS TO ASK
YOUR DOCTOR

Start a Chemotherapy Notebook. Write everything down. Take your list of questions with you for each doctor's appointment. Designate some of your notebook pages for writing your observations about your physical and emotional responses to the drugs, to the administration of the drugs, to your waiting-room experiences. Writing helps. A written record helps you distance yourself from the fears we all have when we sign up for these unknowns. Here are some questions to ask your doctor to get you started. You will think of some of your own to add to this list:

1. What drugs will you be giving me and how do they help?
2. Am I on an experimental program? Am I a guinea pig?
3. How successful is this treatment for the type of cancer I have?
4. When will my chemo treatments begin?
5. Who will be giving me my treatments?
6. How will they be given?
7. Where will I receive my treatments?
8. How often will I receive my treatments?
9. How long will I need chemo?
10. How can I tell if they are working?
11. How many days will I be sick? How sick?
12. Will I be able to go to work?
13. Does someone need to come with me?
14. What kinds of tests will I need?
15. Can I miss a dose or several doses?
16. Are there any long-term side effects?
17. Will I gain or lose a lot of weight?
18. Will I lose all of my hair?

19. Are there any side effects that I should report right away?
20. Will the drugs affect any children I may have in the future?
21. May I take other medicines while I'm having chemo?
22. May I drink alcohol while on chemo?
23. Will these drugs interfere with my sex life?
24. How much will the treatment cost?
25. Your own questions: _____
26. _____
27. _____
28. _____

Don't plan to ask these questions all at one time. Besides your doctor, you may ask your whole health team—chemo nurse, technician, social worker, dietitian, physical therapist, or pharmacist—about managing chemotherapy.

TOP TEN CHEMOTHERAPY DRUGS: WHAT THEY DO TO CANCER CELLS AND WHAT THEY DO TO YOU

Alkylating Agents

These anticancer drugs have a direct chemical interaction with your cells. They work by stopping or slowing down cell growth.

1. Cytoxan. Used for lymphoma, breast, ovarian, and lung cancer, myeloma, and leukemia. Possible side effects are nausea, vomiting, hair loss, lowered blood counts, blood in urine, and loss of appetite.

2. Alkeran, L-Pam. Used for breast, ovarian, and testicular cancer and myeloma. Possible side effects are nausea and lowered blood counts.

Antimetabolites

These anticancer drugs resemble nutrients that a cell needs to grow. They mimic normal nutrients so closely that they are taken up by the cell by mistake. Once they get inside the cell, they interfere with the dividing process and prevent cell growth.

3. 5-FU (fluorouracil). Used for colon, breast, ovarian, prostatic, gastric, and pancreatic cancer. Possible side effects are nausea, vomiting, diarrhea, lowered blood counts, mouth sores, loss of coordination, skin darkening, and hair loss.

4. Methotrexate. Used for breast, cervical, head and neck cancer, sarcomas, acute leukemia, lymphoma, and choriocarcinoma. Possible side effects are nausea, diarrhea, mouth sores, lowered blood counts, and skin rash.

Anticancer Antibiotics

These are anticancer drugs that come from soil fungi. They are believed to act by blocking cell growth.

5. Adriamycin. Used for breast, lung, thyroid, ovarian, bladder, and testicular cancer, acute leukemias, sarcomas, lymphomas, and Hodgkin's disease, Possible side effects are total hair loss, nausea, vomiting, lowered blood counts, red urine, and mouth sores.

6. Blenoxane ("Bleo"). Used for head and neck, cervical, kidney, testicular, and skin cancer, Hodgkin's disease, lymphomas, and acute leukemias. Possible side effects are nausea, vomiting, mouth sores, hair loss, and red urine.

7. Mutamycin. Used for gastric, pancreatic, colon, and breast cancer. Possible side effects are nausea, vomiting, lowered blood counts, and prolonged loss of appetite.

Plant Products

This anticancer drug involves a chemical from the periwinkle plant. It works by interfering with cell division.

8. Vincristine. Used for Hodgkin's disease, lymphomas, acute leukemias, and breast cancer. Possible side effects are hair loss, constipation, and nerve tingling in fingers and toes.

Hormones

Some forms of cancer respond to hormone treatment, even though it is not yet known how hormones work to destroy cancer cells.

9. Prednisone. Used for lymphomas, Hodgkin's disease, acute leukemias, myeloma, and breast cancer. Possible side effects are increased appetite and sense of well-being, sleeplessness and agitation, fluid retention, acne-like rash, increased blood sugar and blood pressure, stomach and intestinal ulcers, increased susceptibility to infection, increased bruising, and weight gain.

10. Tamoxifen. Used for breast cancer. Possible side effects are nausea and vomiting, hot flashes, vaginal itching and bleeding, headache, and light-headedness.

Other agents

Cisplatin. Used for testicular, ovarian, head and neck, bladder, and prostatic cancer. Possible side effects are nausea and vomiting, ringing in the ears, and dulling or loss of sensation in arms and legs.

TOP TEN SIDE EFFECTS: WHAT TO DO ABOUT THEM

1. Nausea and Vomiting. Respect your feelings! Eat what sounds and feels good to you, especially high protein and high carbohydrate foods. Eat small portions as often as you can. Increase fluids between meals. Drink milk shakes if you have difficulty with solids.

2. Weight Loss. Eat pasta and other high carbohydrate foods. Drink shakes and malts. Learn to snack—carry nuts, dried fruit, and food supplements with you. Read "Top Ten Tips for Adding Calories to Your Daily Diet," on page 104.

3. Mouth Sores. Make your own mouth rinse with warm water, salt, and baking soda. Eat soft, mushy, wet foods. Avoid alcohol, mouthwashes containing alcohol, and spicy foods.

4. Hair Loss or Thinning. It's temporary! Cover your head with a scarf, hat, or wig.

5. Numbness or Tingling Fingers and Toes. Protect your hands and feet. Wear mitts when cooking, gloves when gardening, and heavy socks when out in cold weather. Don't go barefoot. Report to your doctor for possible reduction in dosage.

6. Insomnia. Increase exercise. Learn some relaxation exercises. Avoid daytime naps. Take a warm bath at bedtime; massage and sex work even better.

7. Constipation. Increase fluids. Eat more bran, fiber, and whole grains. Allow time for each bowel movement. Take Metamucil if diet changes aren't working.

8. Diarrhea. Increase fluids to replace fluids lost. Report to nurse or doctor if it lasts more than a day.

9. Irregular Menstruation and Sterility. If you intend to have children, consult with your doctor about birth control and the use of a sperm bank before you start chemo.

10. Libido (Sexual Desire). Talking about your feelings with your partner helps most. Lack of desire is often related to depression. Ask your doctor, nurse, or social worker for sexuality counseling. See pages 138–39.

EAT WELL!

• Chemo patients who eat well during treatment periods are better able to stand the side effects of the treatments.
• Chemo patients who eat well have fewer infections.
• Chemo patients who eat well can maintain their strength and prevent body tissues from breaking down; they can also help rebuild the normal tissues that have been affected by chemo.

For chemotherapy patients, eating well means the following:

• High protein—for growth and repair of cells
• High calories—for weight maintenance and strength
• A well-balanced diet to include the four basic food groups every day (see pages 139–40)

High Protein

During chemotherapy, an increase from 45 to 55 grams of protein to 80 to 100 is recommended. If you're like me, you've heard of calorie counters ever since you were a teenager, but how on earth do you measure grams of protein? Here are some examples:

Hamburger (cooked quarter-pounder) = 21 grams
Tuna (3 oz.) = 21 grams
Cheese (1 oz.) = 7 grams
Egg (one) = 7 grams

Milk (one cup) = 8 grams
Wheat germ (1 oz.) = 9 grams
Yogurt, sour cream (one cup) = 8 grams
Bread (one serving) = 2 or 3 grams
Peanut butter sandwich = 24 grams;
    plus a glass of milk = 32

Ten Tips for Adding Protein to Your Daily Diet

1. Double the strength of milk by combining whole milk with powdered skim milk. Mix one quart of milk plus one cup powdered skim milk, blend, and chill. Double-strength milk can be used in cooking and for drinking.

2. Prepare omelets with double-strength milk, cheese, butter, mayonnaise, wheat germ, and meat.

3. Prepare casseroles with double-strength milk, eggs, butter, mayonnaise, wheat germ, and cheese.

4. Snack on yogurt or puddings made with double-strength milk.

5. Snack on cheese, peanut butter, and crackers.

6. Add wheat germ to cereals, yogurt, and baked goods.

7. Make and eat dessert recipes with a lot of eggs—for example, angel food cake, rice pudding, custard, and cheese-cake.

8. Use double-strength milk to make soups and cocoa.

9. Add grated cheese or chunks of cheese to sauces, vegetables, and soup.

10. Add chick peas, kidney beans, and tofu or meat, fish, eggs, and nuts to salads.

Ten Tips for Adding Calories to Your Daily Diet

1. Add a teaspoon of butter or margarine (45 calories) to your soups, vegetables, potatoes, cooked cereal, and rice.

2. Add mayonnaise (100 calories per tablespoon) to your salads, eggs, and sandwiches.

3. Use peanut butter (90 calories per tablespoon) on apple slices, banana, or celery.

4. Spread honey (60 calories per tablespoon) on your toast; use it as a sweetener in your coffee or tea.

5. Add sour cream (70 calories per tablespoon) to yogurt, vegetables, fresh fruits, raw vegetables, and salads.

6. Put whipping cream (60 calories per tablespoon) on yogurt, fruit, puddings, hot chocolate, and Jell-O.

7. Make fruit juice shakes—one cup vanilla ice cream, one cup apricot nectar, and two teaspoons raspberry syrup.

8. Drink fruit nectars.

9. Add raisins, dates, and chopped nuts to hot and cold cereals.

10. Carry snacks with you: nuts, dried fruits, crackers and cheese, granola, and chocolate.

More Help for Nutrition

Call the toll-free 800 National Cancer Institute number, page 111, and ask for a free single copy of *Eating Hints: Recipes and Tips for Better Nutrition during Cancer Treatment* (NIH Publication No. 83-2079).

CHEMO TALK

Here is a glossary for chemo talk. Its purpose is to help you understand some of the technical terms you will read and hear about so that you'll be able to communicate more easily with your health team. Look over the list so that you'll feel comfortable when you hear the words. Remember, too, that when the word has to do with you and cancer, your level of anxiety is higher, and it's hard to remember unfamiliar terms.

For example, I can never remember what *metastasis* means or how to say it!

Adjuvant chemotherapy: The use of drugs to treat cancer after surgery or radiation.

Alopecia: Hair loss from the body and/or scalp.

Anemia: Low red blood cell count; symptoms include shortness of breath, lack of energy, and fatigue.

Anorexia: Absence or loss of appetite for food.

Antiemetic: A medicine that prevents or controls vomiting.

Antineoplastic: Preventing the development, growth, and spread of cancerous cells.

Benign tumor: A noncancerous growth that does not spread to other parts of the body.

Blood count: The number of red blood cells, white cells, and platelets in a given sample of blood.

Bone marrow: The inner, spongy tissue of a bone where red blood cells, white cells, and platelets are formed.

Cancer: A general name for over one hundred diseases in which abnormal cells grow out of control; a malignant tumor.

Catheter: A tube used for the injection or withdrawal of fluid.

Cell: The basic structure of living tissues; all plants and animals are made up of one or more cells.

Chemotherapy: The treatment of disease with drugs.

Clinical trial: Research studies conducted with patients to evaluate a new cancer treatment, also called experimental chemotherapy.

Combination chemotherapy: The use of several drugs at the same time or in a particular order to treat cancer.

Estrogen: The primary female sex hormones. Synthetic estrogens are used in the treatment of some cancers.

Experimental chemotherapy: *See* Clinical trial.

Gastrointestinal (GI): Having to do with the digestive tract, which includes the mouth, throat, esophagus, stomach, small and large intestine, and rectum.

Infusion: The process of putting fluids (including chemo medicines) into the vein by letting them drip slowly through a tube.

Injection: The use of a syringe to "push" fluids into the body; often called a "shot."

Intramuscular (IM): Within or into a muscle; some anticancer drugs are given by IM injection.

Intravenous (IV): Within or into a vein; anticancer drugs are often given by IV injection or infusion.

Investigational new drug: A drug licensed by the Food and Drug Administration (FDA) for use in clinical trials (experimental) but not approved at the time by the FDA for commercial marketing.

Lesion: Groups of cells that can be solid, semisolid, inflammatory, benign, or malignant.

Libido: Sexual desire and energy.

Lymph nodes: Part of the lymphatic system that helps produce some of the white blood cells and antibodies that defend the body against infection.

Malignant growth: A tumor made up of cancerous cells.

Metastasis: The migration of cancer cells from their original site to another part of the body through the blood and lymph vessels.

Neoplasm: A tumor or abnormal new growth or swelling of tissue.

Nodule: A small mass of tissue, usually malignant.

Oncologist: A doctor who is a cancer specialist.

Oral medication: The process of taking anticancer drugs by mouth.

Palliative: A treatment that eases without curing, i.e., one that shrinks the cancer to make the patient more comfortable.

Pathologist: A doctor trained to study cells and tissues to determine if a disease is present.

Platelet: A component of blood that aids in clotting. A reduction in platelets can lead to bleeding or bruising.

Prognosis: The prediction for the outcome of disease.

Protocol: The plan for experimental or clinical trial treatment.

Radiation therapy or radiotherapy: Cancer treatment with radiation (high-energy radiation from X-ray machines, cobalt, radium, neutrons, or other types of cell-destroying radiation).

Red blood cells: Cells that supply oxygen to tissues throughout the body.

Regression: Shrinkage of cancer growth.

Remission: The disappearance of signs and symptoms of disease.

Scans: The computerized pictures of an organ or part of the body such as bones, liver, or brain.

Side effects: Reactions to drugs that are usually temporary and reversible. Not related to drug effectiveness.

Staging: Methods used to evaluate the extent of a patient's disease.

Standard treatment: A cancer treatment proved effective on the basis of past studies.

Stomatitis: Sores on the inside lining of the mouth.

Symptom: A sign or indicator of disease or change in an organism.

Tumor: An abnormal growth of cells or tissues; tumors may be benign (noncancerous) or malignant (cancerous).

Toxic reaction: Dramatic reactions or side effects from drugs.

White blood cells: The blood cells responsible for fighting infection.

HELP WITH CHILDREN

Your children will get their clues from you about how to manage family living with a parent with cancer. You are the expert on your own children. Trust yourself with what feels right in helping them understand and deal with cancer and chemotherapy in the family.

Other chemotherapy parents with young children have devised ways that work best for them. Here are some of their special considerations and principles that may help you:

• Be sure that your children hear about cancer directly from you, not by accident from someone else.

• Informed children are trusting children.

• Your child has a right to know about cancer in the family.

• A good time to tell your children is as soon as you are diagnosed and know how you are going to be treated. Answer all questions as simply as you know how. Don't tell them more than they want to know. Don't lie or make promises you can't keep. Don't frighten them with test results not yet in, financial worries, or things no one can control.

• Admit your sadness, fear, and anger to your children. Give them permission to feel scary emotions, too.

• Work out daily family living together. Be a team, with all helping as they can. No child two or more years old is too young to help the family in its crisis.

• Continue the home rules and regulations as best you can. Don't let your guilt about being sick break down discipline, a breakdown that will be more unsettling to your children. This is a time when many children act out more than usual because they miss the attention they usually had before the illness. Be creative about finding other adults in the family or friends to spend extra time with the children.

Any family crisis, even cancer, provides an opportunity for the family to grow and share the emotional burden. Look for resources within your family that strengthen the bond between its members. It's a good time for parents to teach children that it's true that life is hard. And just as they learn how hard it is, they can learn, too, that life is worth living by the good feelings they get from their parents, who are proud because the children are managing so well with a major crisis in the family—a parent with cancer.

CANCER SUPPORT GROUPS

American Cancer Society, 777 Third Avenue, New York, NY 10017; telephone: (212) 736–3030. Or better yet, look in your local phone book in the white or yellow pages (under cancer) for your local or state cancer society. Depending on where you live, there are several programs. For example, CanSurmount is a patient visitation program in the hospital; I Can Cope is a support group for the patient and family outside the hospital; Road to Recovery is a transportation program to get patients to and from their treatment; and Reach for Recovery is a breast cancer program. Find out how your local cancer society can help you through these programs and more.

Cancer Care, Inc., National Cancer Foundation, 1 Park Avenue, New York, NY 10016; telephone: (212) 679–5700. A New York metropolitan area social service agency, Cancer Care provides counseling, home health care, volunteer visitors, and financial assistance for cancer patients and families.

Candlelighters, a support group for parents of children with cancer: 123 C Street, SE, Washington, DC 20003; telephone: (202) 659–5136 It has over one hundred chapters, worldwide, providing emotional support and education.

National Cancer Institute, a U.S. government agency, is part of the National Institutes of Health (NIH). Our tax dollars provide the services; probably the most helpful is the toll-free help line:

1-800-4-CANCER

I've tried it. It works! You can count on personalized answers to your cancer-related questions by dialing this toll-free number. A trained staff member of the Cancer Information Service will provide you with the latest facts on all types of cancer, using information updated by the National Cancer Institute. The first things you may want to find out are what are your local cancer support groups, what are your local cancer resources, where are the approved cancer hospital programs. Besides the local information you can ask about financial help, descriptions of drugs and their side effects, sexuality counseling, and anything you want to know. This 800 number is good in all states, with the following exceptions: in Hawaii (Oahu), call 805–524–1234 (from neighboring islands, call collect); in Washington, D.C. (and suburbs in Maryland and Virginia), call 202–636–5700; and in Alaska, call 800–636–6070.

In addition, you can ask to have the following free publications mailed to you from the National Cancer Institute.

FREE CHEMOTHERAPY-RELATED PUBLICATIONS

1. *Chemotherapy and You: A Guide to Self-Help during Treatment* (NIH Publication No. 85-1136)

2. *Eating Hints: Recipes and Tips for Better Nutrition during Cancer Treatment* (NIH Publication No. 83-2079)

3. *Taking Time: Support for People with Cancer and the People Who Care about Them* (NIH Publication No. 85-2059)

If you are on chemotherapy, or have a friend or relative on chemo, you will want to have a copy of each of these publications. You can call the toll-free 800 number above or write for free copies to be mailed to you. For more information about particular forms of cancer, its treatment, and possible side effects, write to the Office of Cancer Communications, National Cancer Institute, Building 31, Room 10A18, Bethesda, MD 20205.

Holiday Time

❖❀❖

*I*told my most dramatic hair-loss story to many of my friends a year after it happened. I thought it was a very funny story, mostly because of the surprise element. Many friends laughed with me, but others thought it was more scary than funny. Knowing there've been mixed reviews for this version, and not knowing how your own hair loss experiences compare, I hope this account brings a smile to you.

Sure, people told me I'd lose my hair. I knew it was going to happen. But I don't remember anyone ever telling me how I'd lose my hair. How fast it happens and what it feels like and where it goes. I mean, that's an awful lot of hair to drop in a week. Have you ever had anyone tell you that lost hair ends up mostly in your mouth? On your pillow? Sticking to the back of your nightgown, shirt, sweater? Dropping off in gobs in the sink? Wherever you bend your head? Of course not! People don't tell you useful things like that. They don't tell you to get a hair net to wear at night so that you won't choke on the hair in your mouth. You never get an idea of what to expect. Great big mouthfuls in the middle of the night! Yuck!

Just how important is hair, anyway? Why did the nurse in the chemotherapy workshop at Sloan-Kettering say that "the single most disturbing chemo side effect is hair loss"? Does it really work to take ice packs to the chemo unit and apply them all over the scalp just before the drip is inserted and then the minute after its out, as I saw one young woman do? Will an ice bag on a man's bald spot really bring back hair he didn't have before chemo, as one man told me? I found out in the chemotherapy workshop that it depends on which drugs you are getting and on how strong the dosage is.

I remember well the moment when I first discovered hair loss—one week after my first hit. I was feeling so proud that I had recovered and could eat again, could walk around and work and enjoy life again, that hair loss was furthest from my mind. I didn't look for it in the mirror, or when shampooing my hair. In fact, I had understood that some people lose their hair and that others aren't affected at all. Little did I know that that meant some people who didn't have Adriamycin. All of these big-dose Adriamycin people have total hair loss. Anyway, while visiting a friend for dinner, I excused myself and went to the bathroom. I happened to glance down, and there—in my panties—was a fistful of hair! I did a double take and tried to think what on earth was happening to me when "hair-loss syndrome" flashed on my mental screen. I jumped up from the toilet, panties and slacks around my ankles, short-stepped over to the mirror as fast as I could, and looked at my head. I took a handful of hair, gave a tiny, teeny pull and out came a handful of hair. I did it again. And then once more. Then I looked down. I just couldn't stop testing. I gave a little pull. That came out too! Oh my God! Did anyone in this world tell me, did I read anywhere, did anyone even intimate that you lose your hair everywhere? Even down there? I pulled myself together and went home and rushed to the booklet the nurse had given me about the side effects of chemo. I flipped the pages until I found the page with my list of drugs. My eyes shot over to the right of the page to see the list of side effects. There they are: Cytoxan—hair loss; 5-FU—hair loss; Adriamycin—total hair loss. I'd never noticed the word *total* before today.

Starting with the yellow pages and a call to Sloan-Kettering for a recommendation, I ended up, with Lita, across from Bloomingdale's in the wig shop. Lita is my artistic, fashion-wise, French-class friend. With enthusiastic emphasis on the fashion component, she joined me in my search for hair. It was holiday time. The place was bustling. In the window was a bright red-orange nylon wig with a Cleopatra cut: straight line, shoulder length with bangs. Many glamorous women were in the shop wanting another color, another style, another look, a special holiday hair look—something a little different. Here am I wanting hair that's just me—nothing different about it.

Lita was so turned on by the shop that she would gladly have jumped into the wig buyer's chair, facing the whole wall of mirrors, and tried them all on herself. But it was reluctant me who ended up in that chair facing the mirrors, who had to spend the money, and who had to violate her self-image with a wig. But no matter how it felt, it had to be done.

Theresa, the owner of the shop, assured me that she had many chemo clients. She knew just what I wanted, and for $300 there would be nothing to it. When I said I had $50 in mind, she and Lita quickly assured me I'd be happier with something for around $100. I agreed, and she went out to look. A moment later behind me in the mirror I saw in her hands a mass of curly hair, suitable for a seventeen-year-old rock star, about to go on my head.

"Wait a minute," I cried, shooting my hand up over my head. "When I had all my hair, it was one-fourth of that and straight! My hair was thin. I'm small—five feet tall, 110 pounds. I don't want that much hair on my head. Besides, curly hair doesn't look serious. How on earth could I ever sell a book with that thing sitting on top of my head?"

"I'll fix, I'll fix, just let me try . . ."

Detesting the hideous experience, I slid way down in the chair, hoping the abhorrence would disappear from the mirror as Theresa tried to pull me back up by the wig, which, of course, came off to expose my sickly white bald head to the glamorous holiday shoppers.

"Okay, I'll find another one."

Oh, God. I was right in the first place. I should go with the hats and bandanas. I'm just not the type to wear a wig.

The seventh wig came with less hair, no curl, and, I must admit, exactly the color of my hair. I agreed it was the one for me. Theresa said it was perfect. It just needed a little thinning and trimming. I asked her when she could do it, and she explained that it cost $10 extra. I thought I had already paid $50 extra and said, "No thanks, I cut my own hair to save money, so I guess I can cut my own wig with it right in front of me." And I did.

Parker invited me to his annual "pass along" Christmas party on December 13. I've no better friend than Parker. Still, I had mixed feelings about going to that year's Christmas party. He had invited me every year since my move to New York City. It's his traditional party, with the same close friends who take along gifts they were given last Christmas and want to "pass along" to someone else. It's the most elegant party I go to. By far. Among the guests are Arnold Scaasi, Louise Nevelson, several editors from sophisticated magazines, a sprinkling of French people to give an international flavor, and Park Avenue couples from old-money families. I hesitated. All of those fashionable people there! They're so different from the academics I'm used to in Vermont, or the feminists I work with in Boston, or the not-for-profit others I tend to spend my time with in New York. They are so involved with looks, in ways I don't even see, much less know or understand. With all of that emphasis on looks, what on earth will I do without hair, and with my hundred-dollar wig?

Well, knowing Parker and how he loves me, I finally figured out I couldn't go wrong. Besides, Louise Nevelson wears outrageous hats. I had seen her in a riding hat at an art gallery opening and in a wool toque pulled way down over her head in a restaurant, so why not pretend I chose to wear a hat to the Christmas party?

I decided my purple hat would be perfect. I'd wear it without the wig, and I'd go to his apartment before the party and check it out in his mirror. Well, when I bought the hat I had a little hair. Now I had none. When I looked in Parker's mirror, the hat came down so low on my head I couldn't see. I thought if I were really tall, it would be okay; I'd just stand there with that hat low over my eyes and look down at everyone. But at five feet and wearing a hat down over my eyes, I'd miss the whole party! Now what will I do? Maybe if I stuff something in the top of the hat? That's it! I'll go get one of Parker's big handkerchiefs, make it into a ball, and put it in the crown, lifting it up off my head by half an inch.

It works! Look—that's just right! Well, hat, handkerchief, and all, here I go . . .

One fascinating person after another. An editor heard me mention New Guinea. Oh, good, I'll talk about New Guinea. Then Parker, always a gracious host, came by and said, "Joyce, tell Madalynne about your new cookbook business." So I was off and running about my cookbook business. By the time midnight rolled around, I had tasted each elegant dish, looked over every delicious person, watched the champagne being passed around on silver trays, and, no doubt about it, I felt like a million dollars! Even with no hair. I had risen above it, had once more gotten outside myself, beyond cancer, and been in another dimension with Parker and his friends in New York's Christmas season. It's possible, it's possible. Thank you, Lord, it's possible.

How did I ever get into such a situation for this, of all Christmases? Ned and Elizabeth were both in California, I had hoped Bill was going away, as he had the year before, and I'd have the children at the farm, knowing they didn't want to be in New York. And knowing Bill doesn't care about Christmas. I'm the big Christmas nut in the family. Anyhow, Bill wasn't going anywhere, and I was scheduled for my third hit on December 26. This situation set me up for a very heavy "poor me" feeling. I can't think of many things to add that would have made me feel more as if the world were doing a number on me. Everyone has Christmas plans—or at least everyone with a family and friends. And I have both of those things. But nothing was right. Finally, I decided to write to both kids and ask them whether they would like to spend Christmas with me in the city and go to Vermont the next day. I know that my children do nothing out of a sense of duty, unlike their 1950s parents at that age, so it was safe to ask. They both said coming to New York for Christmas Day would be fine. My whole holiday season changed.

In the end, though, Christmas didn't go as well as I had hoped. Ned had a bad cold, Elizabeth hated the city, and it felt like thirty below zero on Christmas night. I had decided that since they had never been to Radio City Music Hall, it would be a perfect Christmas night event. How wrong can parents, even thinking parents, be? The crowded hall, the glitzy stage show was hardly designed for my nonconformist, laid-back California college students.

Chemo on the twenty-sixth. That will be a piece of cake compared with messing up Christmas night with my children.

The Christmas season made me think through how prayer fits into my life with cancer, especially since so many people tell me, "I'm praying for you." One woman told me I was on her father's prayer list, and I don't even know him. More and more I began to wonder, what does it mean, anyway, when someone is praying for me? After all, I'm hardly praying for myself.

My closest religious friends, the ones with whom I tend to work out religious and spiritual issues, are Lyn and Pat. Pat lives in Boston and is an ordained Presbyterian minister with whom I worked in the days of the women's movement in the early 1970s. Lyn, my Scripture-authority friend, is an Australian physician missionary whom I met in New Guinea and who always urged me to read Scripture. We have stayed in close touch through our letters and a few visits in spite of our living in different hemispheres. Here is my letter about prayer to Lyn:

Dear Lyn,
   If you haven't already read it, I want you to go right out and buy a copy (paperback) of <u>When Bad Things Happen to Good People,</u> by H. S. Kushner. Like you, he knows Scripture. Unlike you, Kushner doesn't think that God personally intervenes for each of us. He doesn't expect God to take the disaster away if people only pray enough or have enough faith. I can't relate, either, to personal intervention prayers that would make everything "right" for me—such as asking God for a clear biopsy, or a long life, or no divorce. To me, "God is good" doesn't mean good to me for what I want within my limited understanding. "God is good" means that if I pray hard enough, I can get in touch with God, who will in turn

*give me courage and strength to handle the particular
disaster, such as cancer or an early death. And if I
believe, God will speak to me through my friends,
through other children of God. In other words, as I
comfort and encourage others, I will be comforted and
encouraged. So it turns out, I do understand prayer after
all, and what others are saying to me when they pray for
me. They mean that, as a spiritual group, we will share
the burden of cancer, the loss of good health, the lousy
bad luck, and the injustices in life together. This time for
me, but next time for another. Amen and love, Lyn. Now
I can say thanks for your prayers!*

Joyce

The Reverend Patricia Budd Kepler is my social-justice
friend. She was on the Harvard Divinity School faculty when
I was NOW's national coordinator for women and religion.
Her favorite issue has always been the inclusivity of women
in the concept of God. Her project at the moment was urban
ministry. Pat is also a filmmaker, and she came to New York
City to get me on video, even in a wig. I consider that true
friendship on my part. Here is my letter to her:

Hi Dear Pat:
   *The church continues to be my community in need.
When I miss a Sunday because of chemo, friends call,
and when I am there, several come to me to ask how I'm
doing.*
   *The Bible classes are exceptionally wonderful, taught
by a very young, just graduated Union theological
student, Heidi Hudnut, the daughter and granddaughter
of well-known Presbyterian ministers. She is very
academic and always does her homework to teach us
about Israel's history, the prophets, the Gospel, the*

parables—the works. No matter how varied our class experience, or how little some of us know, like a good teacher, she always finds something encouraging to say to each person. You'd love her, Pat, and be proud that she's a sister in your church. And, of course, she knows of your feminist theology work. You'll be pleased to know, Pat, that I add a strong shot of much needed feminism to the Bible class. Two classmates of mine, Etta, in her nineties, and Mary, in her eighties, seem to get a kick out of having an outspoken feminist in their midst.

Pat, I know that having a spiritual community isn't as crucial for everyone as it is for us. Others I have met at Sloan-Kettering have told me that they find support groups in their family, in their work community, through cancer support groups, and in a great variety of places.

Most cancer patients have a family place and a workplace that provide a natural support group. But I felt quite lost without my family when I first moved from Vermont until I found a church, which is my family. My church is known for its community and family concerns. When we pledge money, we pledge our time as well. When we raise money for ourselves (building and program), we raise an equal amount to give to others. Besides that, here in this great big city, right on the Upper East Side, are the best potluck dinners, with more toddlers than I have ever seen in one place.

But, like a family, we have our blind spots. Even though we have women clergy, the church is not working very hard at being inclusive for women in language and concept. Like many churches, it seems to find it difficult to be concerned with justice for the women sitting right in its pews. Probably part of the problem is that I have yet to meet another person there who is concerned with feminist issues. Since I've had cancer, I notice that social justice is not uppermost in my mind. When I win this chemo battle, I must get back to those other important battles of life.

What seems to concern me most right now is prayer and cancer. I have come to the conclusion—for now, anyway—that it doesn't make sense to ask to be cured of cancer, because I don't think God intervenes in a personal way against the laws of nature. If God did so, why would some be cured and others not? The world is so full of injustice that to act as if God could intervene for me while injustice still rages toward others just doesn't make sense to me. Even as I write this, I know you pray for healing, and I want you to tell me more about what you expect from your healing prayer services.

But I do want to talk to God as I go along. I need the conversation that brings God's presence into focus on my issues. Along with Rabbi Kushner and the Reverend Heidi Hudnut, I do believe that our Judeo-Christian God is a suffering God as well as a God of an abundant life. Just look at the history of God in the Old Testament and of Jesus on the cross! And if God is a suffering God, then I feel that I am not hit by suffering or bad luck or cancer standing here by myself. Alone. When disaster hits me, God cries for and with me. When disaster hits me, I become very aware of God's other children who comfort me. I believe that God comforts me through others: She speaks to me when you speak to me. And I'm for that.

Write and tell me what you think, Pat. You know how your creative mind sparks new perceptions in me.

Much love,
Joyce

December 26. After the dreaded finger prick to count the white blood cells, I went into the women's room. A small, black woman in her forties was standing at the sink and reaching for a paper towel with a big smile on her face. "I'm finished," she beamed.

"I'm just starting," I replied.

"Is this your first time?" she asked.

"I've had two."

The woman continued, "My six months are over—I mean, I'm done!" And then I realized she meant finished—the end, not just for today. "Congratulations!" It was the first time I had ever realized that there will be an end to chemotherapy. From the joy of that woman's talk, from the lilt of her walk, and from the smile from her innermost self, I knew it was a worthwhile time to count on.

The chemo nurse just outside the chemo unit read the blood count and said, "Not today. Your white blood count is down. You'll have to wait a week and see if it goes up."

"Blood count is down? What does that mean? What can I do to get it up? What can I eat that helps? Will I get a cold easily? Will other diseases find their way into me because my immunity is down?"

"What it means is that the chemo drugs you received have lowered your white count below 3 and that you are at a high risk for infection and should take precautions to prevent it. Signs of infection that you should look for and report to me right away are a fever of over a hundred degrees; chills; sweating, especially at night; loose bowels; a burning feeling when urinating; or a severe cough or sore throat. Do not use aspirin or any other medicine to reduce fever unless you check with me first."

Fever over a hundred! Well, I guess I'll know if that happens. No wonder I dreaded chemo. You just never know which is worse: to have the hit or to run around with no white blood cells to fight infection. Anyway, I half listened to the steps the chemo nurse said are important to take to prevent infection when my white blood count is low:

- Avoid crowds.
- Take a shower every day; wash your hands after eating and using the bathroom.
- Use lotion or oil to soften dry skin so that it won't crack.
- Use an electric shaver rather than a razor for shaving.
- Avoid sick people and those with a cold.

I added "Eat well and get your sleep" to her list.

What it really means to me to have a low blood count and no chemo today is that I need New Year's plans. More holiday plans. I was going to be down and out with chemo and didn't have to think about it, but now I'll have the chemo after New Year's. What's everybody else going to do? Ned and Elizabeth have gone back to California. Betsy is in Vermont. Lita is in Connecticut. Ann is in Arkansas. . . . I know: I'll call Beverly. She was my favorite housemate from my single teaching days of thirty years ago, and my Parisian roommate the first year I was divorced. She's my age but looks to be in her early forties, and she still has her Boston accent. She's the most attractive friend I've got. Her cheerfulness and love of teaching French to teenagers make me feel good.

We decided I'd take the train and she'd meet me in Westport and pick a place for New Year's Eve lunch. She knows I love to take the train, so out I went. I had on my purple hat. After Parker's party, I decided that it was so good-looking that I'd even wear it when I do have hair. Beverly wanted to see my new wig right away. I had brought it in my bag to show her, so after lunch I gave her a style show of the latest in hundred-dollar wigs. However, Beverly didn't go along with my joking about anything as crucial as hair and said, "Joyce, I'm giving you ten dollars for your Christmas present to take that wig in and get it thinned and cut so you'll wear it."

That very day—New Year's Eve—I rushed to the wig

store. You can imagine the brisk business they were doing, but, oh yes, for a chemo patient, they would thin and trim the wig and have it ready for New Year's Eve.

What a difference! As I sat in the Oyster Bar at the Plaza a couple of hours later, eating Wellfleet oysters on the half shell, I looked in the mirror behind the bar and saw that Beverly was right. This wig works. It's me in that mirror right over there.

The Last
Big Hit

◇❀◇

Even though it had been a month since I'd last seen Dr. Minelli, when I went in to be checked and to get the prescription for my last big hit, I was still very angry with him. I wanted to know how it happened that I had to learn from the pharmacist and the nurse that the last antinausea prescriptions—for Thorazine and for Reglan— weren't compatible. How could he prescribe oral Reglan, to be taken when I got home, when I couldn't possibly keep it down? Even worse, what kind of doctor would prescribe two drugs that didn't mix with my central nervous system? He explained that Reglan works for most people. Then I was even angrier. Why would he prescribe for "most people" when I was right there in front of him and telling him about my particular reactions: throwing up for twenty-four to thirty-six hours even with the prescribed antinausea Compazine taken by shot and suppository; telling him that if I drink one drink too many, or eat too much, or am in a car with someone smoking, I always throw up? I have a toxic response to too much alcohol and drugs of any kind. Obviously, my body wants to rid itself of these chemicals; it doesn't tolerate foreign substances. Knowing that, I would think it might be better not to take any more drugs, not even so called antinausea drugs. Other people must have experienced the same thing.

He muttered something, and I responded, "You just don't think things through! All you care about is the main event of chemotherapy. You don't give a damn about the side effects. And if attitude makes a difference, a lot more thought would be worthwhile for helping patients handle side effects."

There. I had gotten that out of my system. There's always that imbalance of power between doctor and patient. After all, I'm dependent on this guy! He could say, "Go get another doctor if you don't like the way I do business," or not answer any further questions, or send in the residents and fellows instead of following my case himself. And, of course, he might not make himself available if I have another recurrence a few years from now. Realizing the risk, I said it all anyway. Luckily for me, he stayed with my case: I certainly didn't want to start with somebody new.

January 3. I've got a big reward coming up—the reward for getting through "the big three" before starting the piece-of-cake phase of every week with much lower dosage. Going in for the third hit, I thought that the sooner I got to celebrate the end of the first phase, the better. And I decided I'd go to Key West so that I'd really know I was celebrating.

I felt that with each hit I needed a different friend and approach. Lita came with me this time and brought along

Eudora Welty's short stories. If I had to wait for someone to teach me relaxation techniques, my three hits would be over. Some of you will be familiar with the different ways to relax before and during chemo. The theory is that if you can relax, you can reduce your anxiety and the nausea that precedes chemo in some patients, making the whole procedure easier for you to take. The main relaxation techniques are the following:

• **Tension Relaxation.** Take a deep breath and tense a particular muscle or group of muscles. For example, squeeze your eyes shut or clench your fist. Hold your breath, and then let go and feel your tension draining.

• **Rhythm.** Take deep breaths, keeping a slow rhythm. Lung cancer patients must check first with their doctor before trying deep-breathing exercises. Say to yourself, "In, one, two. Out, one, two." Relax and go limp each time you breathe out.

• **Imagery.** A daydream that uses all your senses. Starting with your eyes closed, breathe slowly and relax. Concentrate on breathing; then imagine a white light ball of healing energy, or the white angels like the ones my Vermont friend Annette called on, or something bright blue, the healing color. Move the healing energy to the tension part of your body, and ask it to lift out the pain or discomfort. Imagine the ball or angels taking the pain and tension away as you breathe out, and coming back in to get more when you breathe in.

• **Distraction.** Watching television, doing needlework, building models, or my favorite, bringing a friend along to chemo to read a story are all ways of losing yourself to keep you from thinking of pain at home or the possibility of another slipped needle.

• **Biofeedback.** Special machines can help you control

your heart rate, blood pressure, and muscle tension. Your nurse can refer you to someone to teach you biofeedback.

• **Hypnosis.** Some patients learn self-hypnosis, like the man from my church who goes into a trance off the edge of his childhood sliding chute. Again, your nurse can refer you to someone trained in this method if you want to give it a try.

Distraction seems to be my best relaxation technique. Up to my old "denial tricks," I know I can relax with a good story. I can get out of myself—beyond the drip—on a good Eudora Welty story almost anytime.

But before Eudora and after Dr. Minelli, I met the nurse who routinely (though always personally) asked how things went the last time. When I responded that I felt stronger between each bout of throwing up for my second twenty-four hours, she was aghast. "Twenty-four hours! Most people don't vomit more than four to six hours." I had assumed that because people tell how terrible it is they had the same twenty-four-hour reaction that I had. After all, who would complain with a lousy four to six hours of throwing up? You would hardly be weak after four to six hours, because you wouldn't go without eating for two or three days. Anyway, the nurse wanted to know how I responded to Decadron.

"Decadron? I've never had it."

"You've never had it? That's the problem! It's wonderful. There isn't anything else like it. It's the very best antinausea there is, and it works for the largest number of people. Wait right here! I'm going to run and ask Dr. Minelli if he'll write a prescription for you."

Dr. Minelli sauntered in. "Try it," he said, and sauntered out.

God! I'm thrilled. Aren't I lucky to have drawn this particular nurse, who really knows about antinausea? It was dripped in along with the chemo drugs, and I hardly knew where I was, as Lita sat on a little stool close by and began reading, "Mrs. Watts and Mrs. Carson were both in the post office in Victory when the letter came from the Ellisville Institute for the Feeble-Minded of Mississippi . . . ," the story according to Eudora Welty. Well, I must admit I noticed the Cytoxan opening my nasal passages with its cold metallic sensation, and I watched every drop of the bright red Adriamycin come out of the syringe and into my hand. But after that I leaned back in the leather chair thinking about that new antinausea miracle, losing my anger at Dr. Minelli for not paying attention to nausea side effects. "Aimee Slocum," continued Lita, "with her hand still full of mail, ran out in front and handed it straight to Mrs. Watts, and they all three read it together. . . ."

At home on Thursday night, I was poised for the usual buildup at around nine o'clock, then at eleven o'clock. Time for bed, and nothing happened. I've found the solution. Thank you, nurse! Thank you, Decadron! Thank you, Dr. Minelli; for agreeing to give it a try even after my confrontation.

Oh no! Run! Made it to the bathroom. What time is it? It's five o'clock on Friday morning. I started my twenty-four-hour siege of vomiting, exactly six hours later than usual. When my friends appeared Sunday night to cheer me up and see if I had survived the last hit, I couldn't get out of bed. The publishing appointments I had made for the Tuesday after the Thursday chemo, I now had to cancel. On Wednesday the world still smelled indescribably awful. It made me sick (gave me the shudders) just to think of most foods, and I couldn't keep those food thoughts out of my mind. So much for Decadron.

Am I complaining? I don't want to be—after all, I've just survived the three big hits. I'm well enough to take off for

Key West and see the tropical flowers, feel the soft warm breezes, eat fish, and see, see, see.

When there are as many unknowns as chemotherapy presents, people make up their own anxiety control program. Mystery and magic abound to deal with chemotherapy. One of my favorite stories about dealing with side effects by reducing anxiety is from my Hardwick Junior High School friend Annette, who lives now in Ohio. She was on chemo for eighteen months, a length of time hard for me to imagine. Knowing that she faced a long-term program, she had studied several relaxation techniques and had learned to imagine the chemo drugs going into her system and fighting her cancer cells in this way. She imagined herself lying on the hot white sand of Pawleys Island, in South Carolina, and seeing a flock of white sea gulls. As she looked at the sea gulls, they turned into angels, who came to her to ask how they could help. She told them to take control and to attack the cancer cells. Then she could stand back, relaxed and confident that the angels were there—that they were in total control. She didn't need to worry; they would kill off the cancer cells.

This worked so well for Annette that she decided to call on her angels when she had sleeping problems, which is a common side effect of many chemo drugs. She often woke up in the middle of the night with painful hands and numbness in her arms and wrists. It was a reaction of her chemotherapy, called carpal tunnel syndrome, a cutting off of circulation. She even had to wear hand braces at night to keep her hands open and the blood circulating. When nothing else worked, she called on her angels and found imagery to be her most effective response.

I asked my school friend what helped most in this life-threatening crisis: there she was with three daughters who had left home, in the midst of a separation that would surely become a divorce after thirty years of marriage, not a hair on her head, and braces on her hands at night. She quickly replied, "Three things: prayer, my angels, and a job."

"You got a job?" I quickly replied, knowing more about the world of work than the world of angels.

"Yes! I started working two to three days a week as a dental hygienist, after not having had a paid job in twenty-five years. My new job provides exactly what I need most—new friends and a network of very supportive women who know what life is like for me."

Once again, there's that search for a support group in the midst of a cancer crisis. For me, friends and church provide a family; for others, the workplace does. Still others prefer to be in a cancer support group where everyone knows what it's like to go through this dreadful experience.

Here's how a man from my church managed his chemo stress. Walter told me that the pain in his upper arm during the time he was actually getting the drugs was so bad that he decided to try self-hypnosis to reduce the pain. A friend of his who works in a pain clinic taught him to go right into a hypnotic state that freed him from fear and from side effects. He asked the nurse not to talk to him during the half-hour drip procedure. Walter started his hypnotic state by imagining himself on the sliding chute he used to play on as a toddler. By the time he slid down the steepest part and was ready to go over the edge, he would drop right off into a no-pain state. Walter had problems sleeping and used the same imagery at night to relax, falling asleep from his hypnotic state—all beginning on his trusty boyhood sliding chute!

My management magic was distraction—a friend beside me to dilute the poisons. The worst was now over for me. Or at least that was the promise. I was eager to write Dr. Hellman with a report of what the first phase of chemotherapy was like.

January 9, 1985

Dear Sam,

I survived (just barely) my big three hits of chemo and am writing to tell you about it, so you'll have more firsthand information about "what it's like."

Both times that I went back for the next round, my blood count was too low, so I waited a fourth week, when it was okay. Dr. Minelli thought it could have been delayed because of my radiation. But I can't imagine a connection between my bone marrow producing white blood cells and radiation of my breast area five years ago. I'd be interested in knowing what you think. My theory is that my cells respond slowly to the drugs, and possibly to cancer, because it took five years for the recurrence. Does that make sense?

I am not a complainer. I'm known as an optimist. And yet everything in my description of chemo suggests that nothing is right with it. What do you think, is this displaced anger? Is the anger at chemo? Or at the injustice of having cancer in the first place? I don't think so. I think more support services built into the chemo process—more written information, a one-page handout in the chemo unit like the one in nuclear medicine, one hour of group work, or access to information from the reception room of the chemo unit—would go a long, long way toward helping us all win the chemo battle. I feel strongly that very little thought is given to side effects or to anything other than the "main event" of the chemo. And if it's true that patients' attitude makes a difference in their recovery, the lack of serious thought about how patients handle chemo just doesn't make sense to me.

When I was last at chemo, I picked up a pamphlet announcing a workshop on chemotherapy. I have called to see if it's for patients or for health care workers, and will attend if possible. If it is for patients, I have to wonder why I didn't know about it, what the outreach is for something like this, and why the doctor (or nurse, for that matter, or Connie) didn't make a point of handing a brochure to each patient in the unit.

I'm looking forward to the "easier" phases.

Yours sincerely,
Joyce

The following week I attended my first Sloan-Kettering workshop, entitled "Understanding Chemotherapy." I got there at just about eleven, when everyone was looking for the best place to sit to learn as much as possible about these awful side effects that we were all living with. Each person received a packet chock-full of materials, mostly booklets from the National Cancer Institute. About sixty people were there—many of them chemo patients with varying degrees of hair and head covers, varying degrees of weight loss or gain, and varying degrees of looking scared. I had decided to go without a head cover. After all, I had just been to Key West and even had some color on my scalp. Besides, we chemo patients were all in this thing together, and most of us knew how vulnerable we felt without hair. Many of us were on our own, although quite a few spouses, other relatives, and friends had come along and asked questions as well.

Knowing the kinds of solid, nutritious food I needed during chemo, I took my own sandwich and was glad I did because the only food offered at lunchtime was sweet coffee cake!

At the time, I thought the presentations were too general

to be really helpful. When patients asked questions, it seemed, the panel too often replied, "You'll have to ask your own doctor." Worst of all was the program's nutrition part, which reminded me of a Woody Allen version of a 1940s sixth-grade nutrition program. The nutritionist showed slides of basic food groups but refused to make any statement on the big patient concerns: alcohol, macrobiotic diet, and vitamin C. All were issues I had been very anxious about when I took my list of questions to Dr. Minelli. I was feeling anxious and angry as the slide presentation continued and as the simple statements kept rolling out of a smiling nutritionist's mouth. When my tolerance threshold was passed, good manners and concern for the presenters were thrown to the winds. A bell went off in my brain and triggered my bald-headed body to shoot up and angrily speak out as if programmed, "I resent being shown slides of a tray of alcoholic drinks, including highballs and Manhattans, which people haven't drunk in twenty years, with the message that we cancer patients can get our sugar and carbohydrate requirements from alcohol! My own chemotherapist tells me that I can't even have one lousy little glass of wine a day, and here you stand, surrounded by medical experts, with a nine-foot screen showing us a tray of drinks, as if you were subsidized by the liquor store business!" Quickly looking to her colleagues for help, she smiled and asked each of us to ask our own doctors about alcohol. But the all-is-well between-patients-and-medical-team spell had been broken. Others in the group jumped up, and, one by one, each of the biggies were brought out: vitamins; what to do if you run out of the chemo you take at home on a weekend; how to tell if chemo works; what chemo does to sex.

I felt that if they'd added a chemo patient to the panel, many of us in the group would have felt more involved with the process.

This workshop didn't start with the nutrition slides. It

began with Dr. Casper, a staff chemotherapist, telling the group about chemotherapy in general and how it works. He said that most of us at the workshop were being treated with "adjuvant chemotherapy," which means that anticancer drugs are used to destroy any cancer cells that may remain after surgery or radiation therapy. Regarding side effects, Dr. Casper told us that there are more than fifty drugs used alone and in various combinations to treat the more than one hundred types of cancer. Therefore, it is hard to predict whether a particular patient will have a specific side effect. In fact, a certain side effect might show up after one treatment but not after the next one.

Dr. Casper informed us that there are two goals of chemotherapy and that patients should know which applies to them: (1) cure of cancer and (2) palliation, which means reducing the tumor or making the person more comfortable for the remaining time that he or she has to live. He said that the patients in the first group ask him how they are going to function while they are getting their chemo and that those in the second asks him what's going to happen to them in terms of pain and suffering. Dr. Casper pointed out that there are so many variables that patients have to ask their doctors about their specifics. There are no generalities, because the two goals of chemotherapy are so different. As a doctor, he feels confident about giving a heavy dose of chemotherapy to patients he is hoping to cure, because the long-term success is worth the short-term misery.

Barbara Bevel, R.N., the next speaker on the panel, told us how the chemotherapy nurse can help patients. She wanted us to think of the chemo nurse as an educator. She has found that many patients think only the doctors can help with the management of side effects. Ms. Bevel wanted to see patients make better use of the nurses, by asking them any question about chemotherapy that occurs to them, especially about its side effects and about the techniques of coping with them. After all, it's usually the nurses who know patients best, thanks to their conversations with them as they administer the drugs. Ms. Bevel went through the top ten side effects (see pages 102–3) and gave suggestions for easing the problems. The most frequently asked questions were about poor appetite, changes in taste, weight loss, fatigue, and nausea. Here are some of the hair questions asked by workshop participants:

• Do ice packs prevent hair loss? Sometimes, depending on the drug and dosage.

• Do all persons lose their hair? No, most lose some but not all of it.

• When does it start to come back? As soon as the particular drug causing hair loss is stopped.

• How fast will I lose it? The rate varies, but sooner than most people would think.

• Will my new hair still be gray? Not always, changes in color and texture are common.

• Do I need a wig? It's best to buy a wig before you need it, when you still have your own hairstyle.

• What do I look for in a wig? That's a personal preference, usually determined by the amount of money you want to spend as well as by the color, texture, and amount of hair and the style.

One of the women stood up and added more to the wig question. She said the easiest way to find out where to buy a wig is to look through the yellow pages of your phone book, to ask the chemo nurse, or to ask another patient who has one that you like. The price range is usually from $50 to $2,000. She was advised not to get natural hair, even if she could afford it, because it takes so much care, and when you're not feeling so hot, you won't feel like all of that work on your wig. The important thing is to like what you buy, so either try to get something just like your own hair or go to the other extreme and make everyone think you've got a new stylist.

Even though there was only one question about sex, both the nurse and the social worker made it clear that many chemo patients were very concerned about their sexual relationships and reproductive possibilities. They wanted us to know that there are health experts at Sloan-Kettering to help us with sexual concerns. It's important to know that not everyone has sexual problems with chemotherapy. But if we do have a problem and want to discuss it, all we have to do is ask.

The main sexual problems that patients bring to counselors involve feelings of inadequacy, feelings of low self-esteem from a change in physical appearances—because of hair loss or breast loss, for example. Another problem is not knowing what to expect on the part of the partner, who often gives the impression of not being interested in sex. As with all sexual problems, talking helps. A common problem for women is vaginal dryness caused by chemo drugs. The best solution is a suppository that provides the proper lubrication. In men, chemo can lower the sperm count. Even though there is no evidence that their libido (sexual desire) is connected to their sperm count, many men report that chemotherapy definitely lowers their interest in sex along with their sperm count. Because anticancer drugs may lower the number of sperm cells, reduce their mobility, or cause other cell abnormalities, couples are urged not to plan conception while the man is undergoing chemotherapy. Men may become infertile as a result of chemotherapy and may want to find out about sperm banking before they begin their chemo.

The chemo nurse cited the main sexual myths that frighten many people. Here are the primary points to remember:

• You cannot "catch" or give cancer through sexual intercourse.

• You cannot "catch" the side effects of chemotherapy through sexual intercourse.

• You cannot get radiated through sexual intercourse.

If, despite the facts, you feel there's a little bit of truth to any of these sexual cancer myths, talk to your chemo health team. If you are worried or just need more information about sex, and it appears there is no one to ask, by all means call the National Cancer Institute (the 800 number is listed on page 111), or call your nearest teaching hospital with a cancer unit and ask to speak to the social worker or nurse in chemotherapy.

After my outburst on alcohol and nutrition, I didn't dare bring up sexual functions. But I thought it funny that not one medical expert felt it important to mention that one good hit of chemo finished my forty-year habit of monthly menstruation. And the unexpected hot flashes that began with chemo seemed much too ordinary to be discussed with cancer experts.

It wasn't because I didn't respect the importance of a nutrition program that I was outraged by the way the alcohol question was presented. After all, good food makes sense for healing. Here's the good stuff the nutritionist gave us.

Most important is eating a balanced diet every day. This includes food from the four basic groups of foods:

1. Fruit and vegetable group. Four servings a day of salads, cooked vegetables, raw or cooked fruits, and juices supply vital vitamins and minerals. A serving can be one-half cup of cooked vegetables, fruit, or juice or one cup or one piece of raw fruit or vegetable.

2. Meat group. Three servings a day of meats, fish, poultry, eggs, or cheese give you proteins as well as many vitamins and minerals. A serving is two ounces of meat, fish, or poultry; two eggs or two ounces of cheese; one cup of dried beans, peas, or nuts; or four tablespoons of peanut butter.

3. Grain groups. Four servings a day of grains and cereals supply a variety of vitamins, minerals, and some protein. A serving is one slice of bread, one cup of cereal, or one-half cup of pasta, rice, or grits.

4. Milk group. Two servings each day of milk or other dairy products provide protein, a variety of vitamins, and, above all, calcium. The following servings supply similar amounts of calcium: one cup of milk or yogurt, one and a half ounces of cheese, one cup of pudding, one and three-quarters cup of ice cream, or two cups of cottage cheese.

The two main messages the nutritionist wanted chemo patients to take home from the workshop were these: (1) Basic good nutrition, using the four groups above plus a high intake of protein, calories, and fluids, is crucial to health care for chemotherapy patients. (2) People have to individualize their nutritional program, taking the best they can from the ideal according to their side effects and their basic eating habits before cancer.

The major concerns that patients express, the nutritionist said, are the issues of alcohol, vitamin supplements, macrobiotic diets, megavitamins, and weight loss and gain. Patients are told to "ask their doctor" about vitamins and alcohol, because the particular drugs they take make a difference in the recommendations. For example, research shows that vitamin C interferes with the action of Methotrexate. The same is true of alcohol. The effects of some drugs, such as Methotrexate, mercaptopurine, Prednisone, and procarbazine, are negated or weakened if mixed with alcohol, and alcohol sometimes produces more-severe side effects.

The research findings on many special diets like macrobiotics are not complete. The value of special diets in treating cancer is unknown.

Weight loss or weight gain is a popular issue, and some patients are afraid of taking Prednisone because they think it will increase their appetite. The point to be made here is that often it's the retention of fluids that causes the weight gain and that as soon as you're off Prednisone, your weight goes back to normal.

The workshop wrap-up was given by the social worker who talked about the impact of cancer on the family. She wanted patients to take home three main points. First, chemotherapy is an individual matter; therefore, the responses to each drug vary as much as persons vary from one to the other. Second, chemotherapy and cancer become a part of who you are. You may be an engineer, a father, a husband; you are also a man living with cancer and coping with chemotherapy. Third, health professionals are available to help you. All you have to do is ask.

Don't be afraid to ask questions. Ask everyone you encounter: the blood count technician, the blood pressure and weight nurse, the chemo nurse, the pharmacist, the physician, the physical therapist, the dietitian, and the social worker.

How to cope with the fear of uncertainty, with the emotional burden that cancer brings to a person, is the most common question put to social workers. This fight with cancer marks the first time many people have faced their own mortality. For spouses and children of cancer patients, it often brings the first perception that their spouse's or parent's life is limited. How to tell children, other relatives, and friends about cancer is another common worry of chemo patients.

After a refreshment break, the participants mingled a little and talked about their response to the workshop and about what else they wanted to know. Several small groups were formed. Its members sat in a circle and shared their chemo-therapy experiences, which focused on frustration with the many unknowns and the attempts to control the uncontrolla-ble: nausea, hair loss, and uncertainty whether or not the chemotherapy is working. There was little talk about cancer. Most of it was about chemo side effects and efforts to man-age them. Many of us went home with the phone number of another chemo patient, someone we could talk to about the horrendous experience we were all undergoing.

It turned out that the workshop provided another way to reach out to others in the same boat. I often met people from my group in the chemo unit. I asked a young man if he got anything out of the workshop. He had never thought of the alcohol and drug mixture before, he told me, and so asked his own oncologist about it that very day.

One woman from my group said she had been having a terrible time with taste bud changes, and the patients in our group made a lot of suggestions—the best one being to eat with plastic instead of silver or stainless knives and forks. Another woman said she had been losing weight rapidly and was sure it was a sign the cancer cells were winning out, until she learned at the workshop that her loss of appetite was due to the drugs she was taking. She immediately made an ap-pointment with the nutritionist to learn how to overcome her loss of appetite and build up her body again.

The middle-aged man next to me told me that until this workshop he had thought he was being used as a guinea pig. He thought that all of us in chemotherapy were on a proto-col, meaning an experimental or clinical trial. When the che-motherapist who started our morning session explained that most of us were on a well-proven, tested, approved combina-tion of drugs for our particular cancer, he felt a lot better about the treatment he was getting. We learned that we couldn't be on an experimental treatment and not know it, because we would have signed a special consent form informing us that we were on such a program. Some of us talked about our options in chemotherapy. Most of us agreed that if the proven methods were not working for us—that is, if our disease continued to progress in spite of chemotherapy—we would be eager to try whatever protocol or experimental program that Sloan-Kettering could cook up. Some of us also agreed that we might not be quite so eager to try experimental treatments outside of a well-known cancer research institution.

If there was one message that all of us took in, it was that it's okay to ask questions, even when the health team appears in a big rush. And we can ask all kinds of specialists: nutritionists about healthful foods, nurses about those mouth sores and nausea, and social workers about our deep worries about our families. Now we've found out it's even okay to worry about sex and learned where to go to for help.

Several months after the workshop, I realized that generalization was better than nothing. At least the issues had become clear: for example, side effects, sexual myths, and sources of further information. Since the first workshop I have met many chemo patients who get their chemotherapy at a doctor's office rather than a hospital or at a hospital without a cancer or education unit. I've talked to many chemo patients whose care has lacked any general health instruction or educational component and who haven't even heard the basic "Eat well!" One man I visited right after his therapy offered me a drink, had one himself, and lit a cigarette. I asked what he had eaten that day, and he said, "Nothing. I lose my appetite with these drugs." When I had asked what his doctor thought of smoking, he said the subject was never mentioned. I couldn't wait to get out of there—my stomach was in a knot from seeing every rule for a healing environment being violated.

I finally learned that an educational program is the exception rather than the rule. In addition to attending several chemotherapy workshops, I interviewed the panels' chemotherapist, nurse, nutritionist, and social worker. In the follow-up interviews I put the following questions to the health professionals: What is the primary message you want the chemo patients to take home with them from the workshop? What are the chief questions chemo patients have been bringing you? If you had more time, what other points would you make that I can add to "The Help Center" for chemo patients? What resources would you highly recommend to chemo patients?

So. Especially for those who have not had the benefit of a chemotherapy workshop, I have compiled the recommended resources and workshop information in "The Help Center," on pages 97–112.

Valentines

◇✿◇

Saturday, February 9, 1985
HAPPY VALENTINE'S DAY, Aunt Eunice

*WHOOOOOOPEEEEE! It worked. I work! I'm really
celebrating today, because my chemo is very
tolerable—for the first time. In fact, I'm just about to try
cross-country skiing in Central Park. I can't believe I'm up
for that.*

*Late Thursday afternoon I had my doctor's
meeting—with Dr. Minelli and two clinical fellows who
are working with him—where the second phase of my
chemotherapy program was explained to me. I will be
taking a new batch of drugs, different from those of my
first three hits. Three of them will be dripped in on the
back of my hand, as in the first phase, and then I'll have
two additional ones to take home and take orally each*

day. The drugs will be in much smaller doses, and once a week instead of once a month, as in my old program.

Ann Williams went with me for my first hit of the second phase. She's my church friend from Arkansas, a lawyer turned stockbroker and the financial adviser in our group. You'll meet her when we come to ski. Ann was eager to see what chemo is like because besides being a good friend to me, she also knows people at work who are on chemo. I'll usually go alone for the hits of this second phase, since I understand they don't have the kick of the first ones. I'll see.

As soon as I got home, I cooked a beef stew for Ann and Betsy. We were all curious how I would respond to this new program and how it would be to live with me in the next three months. I thought I probably wouldn't be eating any beef stew; I certainly didn't want to make the mistake of the first hit! Remember my telling you about the Chinese meal? Do you realize, Aunt Eunice, that I still have an aversion to Chinese food? And when I walk by a Chinese restaurant and get even the smallest whiff of the food, or see rice on a plate, I get the shudders—deep in my soul.

As the early evening went on, I noticed that my body didn't feel the terrible buildup of drugs I had felt before—kind of queasy, but not bad. I couldn't watch TV after my first three hits but could now. We all ate, then watched a great TV show I was feeling well enough to get into. I went to bed about eleven, feeling pretty good and very good about not having thrown up yet—especially watching the clock for that eleven o'clock hour that had always done me in before.

When I got up Friday morning, I felt great but went back to sleep, until 9:30, which is unusual for me. I took my other medications, worked on my College Board

book for about an hour—all routine work on my
computer—then collapsed with absolutely no energy. I
decided that my priority was to stabilize my body as fast
as I could. If little naps helped, it was okay by me. I slept
on and off every few hours, until I had pretty much slept
all day. When I felt as if I were going to be sick—nothing
like the volcanic explosion of the first hit, more like being
carsick—I ate a little something. Carbohydrates and
sweets settled best: like my wonderful oatmeal with maple
syrup or canned fruit. Each time I got past the sickness.
By the time Betsy got home, at seven, I felt very good
and ate a regular dinner. Here I am on Saturday—two
days later—and as good as new.

I just called Ann, and a group of us are going to a
movie tonight, <u>Paris, Texas</u>—written by my favorite, Sam
Shepard, and, I hear, a big hit in Paris, France. I just got
my skis out, and I would say I'm feeling about as well as
anyone could on all of this medication. Getting my skis
out gave me a great boost of energy; I hope it lasts until
I get to the park and back. If it doesn't, I'll just turn
around and walk back home.

Later: I'm back. What a marvelous outing! My first
cross-country ski of the year, cold and sunny and just
beautiful in the park. I've told you how I love running
around the reservoir. Well, in a bigger circle outside the
running track is a bridle path for skiing the two or three
times a year when New York City has snow. The snow
was perfect, and the mere idea that I felt well enough to
be out there was very exciting. I came back to a can of
sardines that you sent me ages ago, Cabot cheese Judy
Daloz brought down, and Vermont maple syrup on ice
cream—quite a Vermont day.

Speaking of Vermont, I'm very eager to get up there
once this winter to see Mrs. Ryder about my cookbook

business and ski Stowe now that I'm all psyched for skiing. The end of February always features the best snow, the warmest sun, and the least number of out-of-staters. How would that work with you?

I'll see my surgeon on February 14 for a regular three-month follow-up. The swimming and ski poling were good for my shoulder, but my hand is swollen, so I'll be glad to see him and find out if there is anything I can do about that. There is such a fine balance between exercising enough to keep the liquids flowing in an arm without lymph nodes and too much, which causes swelling.

Did I tell you I missed my Carnegie Hall concert series three times because of chemotherapy? To be able to go to a concert on Sunday afternoon is my idea of being a real New Yorker, and I'm just learning to like the music. By the feel of today, I don't think I'll be missing anything more. I'll start getting my chemo hits late on Fridays so that Saturday is my only day to laze around and shape up, but without being violently sick—that's nothing to write home about.

Bill called Thursday before my chemo and Friday after it, so he stays in close touch around my chemotherapy trials and tribulations, which is a help.

Thinking of you, and looking forward to my Vermont visit soon,

> *Lots of love,*
> *Joyce*

It was just about this time that the College Board was ready to negotiate a contract for *College to Career*. The editor decided she would like to come by my new apartment and talk about it. It isn't unusual to wear a red bandana with jeans at home, so I figured I was safe: she would never know I didn't have any hair, especially since she didn't know me. The meeting went smoothly until Carolyn asked me to stop by the office to meet the new marketing manager—"You'll like her, Joyce. She's very smart, a young, sharp Harvard M.B.A. with a lot of direct-mail experience, perfect for your new book."

Oh God! What will a sharp marketing manager think of the ideas from someone who wears her hair like this? It's so ordinary. And it looks like a wig. Who at fifty would go around in a wig? It's all the same color. She'll probably think I dye my hair because I'm fifty, so that's why it's all one color. God! She'll probably think my ideas aren't even worth writing down, never mind marketing them with her brand-new Harvard M.B.A. ways to make all kinds of money on my new book that would pay all these doctor bills, and give me weekend trips to Florida and August trips to Paris and let me carry out my three-year-travel plan of Australia, Israel, and China!

Well, here I am. Right in this office to discuss marketing my book with my wig on. Can I look her in the eye? I was as quiet as a little mouse. Does Carolyn, who is new here, wonder why they signed a contract with this nothing-to-say about-her-book person? I have never in my life been quiet and looked down like this when an editor and marketing person, who have already bought my book, are seeking my ideas and enthusiasm in selling it. Looking down? Oh God! Now they'll see the top of the wig. Is this me? With nothing to say about my idea? Why am I acting like this? Is this the same woman who stood up with a bald head at the Sloan-Kettering chemotherapy workshop and told those expert doctors they didn't know what they were talking about? After all, this super M.B.A. is young; how many wigs can she have seen in her lifetime? She probably doesn't even know it's a wig. She just thinks I'm strange for no reason at all! I should never have worn a sweater with this suit; it's so hot in here. Just get me out. . . .

Getting through a weekly routine of chemotherapy in February meant a weekly course of finger pricks. And I was a woman who put off her annual gynecological examination because she couldn't bear the surprise attack of a finger prick. I am talking once a year. Sloan-Kettering's program calls for one every single week—AGONY! The first thing I learned was that it was called a finger stick. The second thing I learned was that there existed a great variety of finger stickers with a wide assortment of techniques. There were small oriental men, big black women, old and young, a Russian, a Hispanic—you name it. America's magnificent array of immigrants for whom English is a second language is reflected in the drawing-blood careers in New York City. Some were outgoing, others very quiet. Trying to guess how to get the "best" (painless) one, the least scary one, wasn't easy! After all, they had a system all figured out. Taking a number from a bakery-shop machine was supposed to line us up with the oriental, black, Hispanic, or Russian: big or little; strong or weak; old or young; slow or very, very fast; English speaking a little bit, a lot; painful or painless.

I remember the time when I tried to get the new technician I'd never seen there before and instead ended up with a HUGE black woman. While she squeezed my finger looking for blood, I imagined her slowly lifting her hand way up above her head as in a good tennis serve, sighting her target, and then—boom!—coming down on my poor tiny, little black-and-blue middle finger, already sore from so many sticks. In reality, I was thrilled when it happened altogether differently. She didn't even lift her arm, just gave this little, gentle push, close to my finger. Painless! Ahhhhhhh. . . . How can I get her next time?

And the third thing I learned was how to change fingers. All of those various blood-drawing immigrants were exactly alike when it came to telling me that they "had" to stick the middle finger (of my right hand only, because the lymph nodes were gone from my left arm; my left arm and hand can never take a stick for blood, a needle for drawing more, or the needle for chemotherapy). That's a lot for the right hand to take, let alone for just one finger, which was bruised within six weeks. Not one to go with the crowd, I gave this situation a lot of thought before coming up with the idea to bandage my right middle finger just before the finger stick. That meant that those technicians had to prick another! After that success, I had it made. With my vulnerable finger bandaged, they learned to stick any old finger, and even my thumb got the finger stick. Relief.

My children felt better when they had detailed information about what I'm taking, so I wrote to them fairly often. At the time of the following letter, Elizabeth had fallen in love for the first time, and her young man had gone to South America to study for a semester.

> *February 12, 1985,*
> *Lincoln's Birthday*

Dear Ned and EDM,
   So glad to have talked to both of you this weekend. And, Elizabeth, I just received your lonesome letter; thanks for it. Missing someone is so hard. But even as I think about it, I know it's the other side of joy with a person. One doesn't feel lonesome unless one loves. And all of it together: loving another person, the joy of being with that person, and the loss when he or she isn't there, and sharing life either together or separately are all a part of intimacy. And intimacy is the most fulfilling experience of life. So I can't wish that you weren't feeling sad;

sadness is the condition of loving. I wish love for everyone, but especially for my children.

I'm writing now to tell you the details about the new drugs I'm on, because I've just looked them all up. You'll see, they're even spelled right! Here they are:

By intravenous (IV) once a week at Sloan-Kettering:

5-FU, an antimetabolite. It resembles nutrients that a cell needs in order to grow. Once taken up by the cell, it interferes with the dividing process and prevents cell growth. Side effects: nausea, vomiting, diarrhea, lowered blood counts, loss of coordination, and loss of hair.

Methotrexate, another antimetabolite. Side effects: nausea, diarrhea, mouth sores, and lowered blood counts.

Vincristine, a plant product derived from the periwinkle plant. It interferes with cell division. Side effects: hair loss, constipation, and nerve tingling and loss of feeling in fingers and toes.

And each day I take the following two orally:

Cytoxan, an alkylating agent. It has a direct chemical interaction with the cells and works by stopping or slowing cell growth. Side effects: nausea, vomiting, hair loss, and loss of appetite. But the effect I feel is a heightened sense of smell, an opening of my nasal and sinus passages (as it was dripped in by IV the first three months); a very cold and metallic smell and taste is in the air—all of the time. I now taste all of this and crave sweets to get rid of it. It makes red meat taste like cold metal. In fact, to show you that it's not my imagination, one man in the waiting room told me he can't even look at silverware anymore and asked his wife to buy plastic knives and forks and to set the table only with plastic while he's on chemo. He told me that he has to eat with plastic to get rid of that bitter metallic taste.

Prednisone, a hormone. It is not known how it works to destroy cells. Side effects: increased appetite and sense

of well-being, sleeplessness, rash, stomach ulcers, and
weight gain.

As you can see, some of these have opposite side
effects, like appetite loss or gain, or constipation or
diarrhea. So I'm hoping they'll cancel themselves out.
Besides, these are possible side effects. Not everyone gets
them, and maybe I won't. I'm not feeling any of them
very much so far. I understand from other patients that
there is a buildup and a cumulative effect causing mouth
sores and tingling fingers and toes. If that gets bad, my
doctor will lower the dosage and then take me off
vincristine completely, because I won't be able to work on
my computer or write. Besides, who would want to lose
the feelings in their fingers? You couldn't get dressed,
never mind write. The positive side effect from
Prednisone that I have felt from the beginning is a sense
of well-being. Lots of energy and a feeling that I'm
going to make it through this chemo business after all.
The nausea is minimal, which is pure heaven for
me.

Ned, I'm sending you the enclosed article from this
month's Atlantic.

Elizabeth, have you turned in your financial aid
application? You haven't mentioned it.

Elizabeth, I am enclosing $100 toward your new
vegetarian board plan—glad it's going well. Good luck on
the Frisbee team!

Muchmuchmuchmuchmuchmuchmuchmuchmuchmuch
LOVE Mom

After three solid weeks of chemotherapy that went well,
I wondered if I could still ski downhill at Stowe. How much
endurance had I lost? What did I have left? What kind of
shape was I in, anyway?

I gathered my friends—even Marylynn from Boston and Ann and Lita from New York—flew People Express to Burlington, and met my aunt Eunice with much excitement. I was back in Vermont, in familiar territory.

Ann had never been on skiis, never been to Vermont; and Lita hadn't skied downhill in ten years. Each one of us got a big bedroom in the house that my great-grandfather had built next to the elementary school in Barre, so his children could come in from the farm and live right next door to a city school.

Bill called as soon as we arrived and wanted to meet us in Stowe so that we could ski together. Bill, Lita, and I spent the day on the familiar Mount Mansfield, where I know all the trails upside down, backward, and forward, having started skiing there in the 1940s. The same wooden T-bar leads to the best intermediate skiing in the world—the Tyrol and Standard trails. I can remember going up there in junior high school with my tall neighbor Billy Rowell and eating a Hershey bar while trying to balance our very different back-end heights on the bar. I remember smoking while riding the T-bar a few years later as a teenager with Peasoup, my French Canadian boyfriend; still later, going up with Bill when I was eight months pregnant; and a few years after that, riding with Ned between my legs, Elizabeth between Bill's legs, with eight skis on the one T. Lots of memories in Stowe on the wooden T-bar.

And here I was adding one more. I took it easy the first time, skiing only half a day. One of the big changes I noticed as a result of chemotherapy was that I would go along expending my energy as always until it was all gone and that on the next day it was still gone! My reserve wasn't there. If I overdid it, it would take me several days to recover. I imagined that's how it must feel to be old: seventies and eighties old, not fifties old, a lot different from young and middle age, when one is in shape and full of resilience. Not wanting to end up all tired out for three days in Vermont, I took the half day of downhill Stowe to see what would happen. Hooray! I felt just fine on Friday and decided I could go for it. I even skied the Nose Dive, my all-time favorite ski trail in the whole wide world. On Sunday our festive group cross-country skied at the famous "Sound of Music" Von Trapp Lodge, to which Judy drove over from St. Johnsbury and where my cousin Mary and my second cousin Laura joined us. We had our own crowd on those trails while the sun streamed through the balsams and pines, casting mottled light patterns on the bright, snowy ground. Friends, beauty, exercise—this is the life.

Spring Break

◇❀◇

"Are you drinking a gallon of liquids a day, excluding coffee and tea? Don't let those chemicals stand in your kidney, liver, or bladder tissues!"

If there is one consistent message from the health team to chemo patients, it's to drink plenty of liquids. "Flush those chemicals out as soon as possible. You know that if you're on Cytoxan it'll crystallize in your bladder." I imagined my bladder—whatever shape and size it is—with black and gray jagged quartz, rocky formations rising up in the lower part of my body like New York's Chrysler Building, thirsting for water with which to get rid of the intrusion.

Proud of my liquid intake—after all, I'd been brought up to drink plenty of Vermont spring water—I didn't anticipate a problem. I mean, does anyone else go to the sink and down a glass of water, just for the health of it? So, planning to triple my usual eight glasses a day, I was totally unprepared when I quickly OD'd on water. What does OD'd on water mean? It means overdosed: you drink so much of it that the very thought of a glass in front of you brings on the shudders.

The search for the perfect liquid, one so good you can drink four quarts of it a day, is a common topic of conversation in the chemo unit waiting room. "What did you drink today? How many glasses could you drink? Did you add lemon, ice, orange, soda, seltzer? One man told me he drank his required quota in Diet Coke. Then someone informed him that the caffeine in Coke is dehydrating, so Coke doesn't count. Someone else said that flat Coke is the answer, especially if you're a little nauseous, because something about it helps settle the stomach. Besides, ice is bad for an upset stomach. Yet another person told me that he was doing fine on twelve to sixteen glasses a day until he learned he wasn't supposed to drink liquids at mealtime, because he was having problems with nausea. One woman told me that as long as she could have unsweetened apple juice or ginger ale after it went flat, she could easily down her twelve glasses.

A teenager said he ate his liquids, in the form of ice cream. A woman right beside him said she did too; she made Jell-O a lot, added extra water, and sipped it all day long. Then there's herb tea, broth, and, of course, beef tea, as New Yorkers call it—bouillon. I found I could drink more very, very weak decaffeinated tea with a little lemon than anything else before OD'ing. And water with a squirt of lemon. But I remember best the time when I found the perfect liquid. I was getting my weekly hit of chemo when the perfect-liquid topic came up in conversation with the woman in the next chair to me. She told me right then and there that there's only one answer to the liquids question—cranberry juice. "Fill your glass almost full of seltzer, add about a fourth of cranberry juice, and you'll never OD on liquids again." I couldn't wait to get home to affirm the perfect liquid. It was my fourth month into chemo, and I was becoming even more compulsive about flushing out those chemicals. I poured my seltzer, measured the cranberry, added a squirt of lemon, and found she was right. It was the perfect liquid— until I OD'd on it just four days later. Like every problem in life, this one doesn't have a perfect solution. The real perfection comes with change. Don't overdo any of them; keep your body guessing so that it can't anticipate and refuse what's coming next. Or at least that's what my body has told me.

My mother has worried about my finances since the day I was divorced. It's just not clear how a writer makes money. It's not like having a husband or a regular job with a salary. Well, she should be worried—I am, too—about my money situation. And yet, most free-lance writers probably don't worry as much as ordinary, salaried people worry about it, or they couldn't be writers.

When we get cancer, its monetary cost seems the least of our problems. Before long, though, cost does become something that most of us have to deal with. Cost sometimes influences our choice of where we get chemo. For example, some insurance plans will pay for chemo only if it is taken as an inpatient in the hospital, while others will pay for an outpatient only in a hospital. Still others will pay for chemotherapy in a doctor's office.

I can remember that the issue of what would happen if I got cancer again was a real problem for me when I first considered getting a divorce. I was aware of losing Bill's terrific university insurance, which paid 100 percent of everything. Insurance plans vary enormously. Many Blue Cross–Blue Shield plans pay 80 percent of the bill, but mine covered only half of the surgeon's bill. Besides, doctors' fees differ a great deal. And the cost of the particular chemo drugs that you get varies even more widely than does the administration of them. I remember one woman telling me that she had to have her $100 up front when she went to her doctor's office in New York City for her weekly chemo hit. When I asked, "But do you have insurance that covers some of that?" she replied, "Oh yes, I get it all back." Needless to say, I didn't come up with much sympathy for her predicament. But I have heard of other patients who get only 80 percent reimbursement, and then there are people like me, whose insurance doesn't cover any of the chemotherapy unless they were inpatients in a hospital. I was charged $75 for the first three hits and $45 a week after that. The charge seemed reasonable to me, after I heard what some others paid.

I've learned that I must have a basic Blue Cross–Blue Shield plan to get into a hospital for surgery. The alternative is to come up with a lump sum of thousands of dollars for admission to the hospital, as do foreigners who come to America for medical treatment. When the bills that are not covered by insurance start to pour in, the hospital or your doctor will usually be satisfied if you agree to pay something on them each month. In other words, make an honest effort to lower your debt with the hospital or doctor. Another point is to negotiate to keep the bills down. Find out if all those expensive tests are necessary and then follow through by doing what you said you would do—pay something each month. I now live as if "the medical debt" were part of my living expenses, just like the rent or the fuel or electric bill.

I decided that if my mother had more information, she wouldn't be quite so worried. Here's my financial statement to her:

March 12, 1985

Dear Mother,
Thanks for your letter and concern about my finances. As you know, I've probably got the least amount of

insurance of any patient at Sloan-Kettering—except for other free-lancers, of course. I have had several meetings about my finances and written a financial letter to each of my doctors just this week. I have agreed to pay $100 a month to the hospital, for outpatient chemotherapy, the cost of which leaps up each week. I should say that they have agreed that that will be okay. And now I have informed each doctor that I will take turns, paying one of them $50 a month. If they've done an excellent job on me so that I live long enough, everyone will eventually get paid. I think that's a pretty fair deal.

I was really lucky to get the $100-a-month arrangement. The hospital kept calling and asking me to pay $1,700 and finally inquired if I would like a financial evaluation. Not sure what that meant, I said sure—although I'd had had an evaluation when I entered the hospital. So two weeks ago, just before my chemo, I went in an hour early, and this very young woman (she couldn't have been over twenty-one) led me through a maze of so-called offices and into a little cubbyhole with no windows or anything. A disconnected phone on an unused desk and some kind of dilapidated copy machine half covered; it looked like a 1920s Aid to Dependent Children's state office in a welfare building.

For some reason I didn't wear my wig and felt especially vulnerable, although I don't usually feel that way at Sloan-Kettering. She asked me about my income. Because I've invested all my money in my cookbook business and don't have a salary, she couldn't understand my situation at all. I could see that I was her first poor writer or not-yet-successful entrepreneur. She kept asking, "Can't you pay that $1,700 in installments?" I tried to explain that I don't have new money coming in at regular intervals, a necessary ingredient for an installment plan agreement. I told Miss Duby I don't know ahead of time *which book ideas I'll sell for how much money, not to mention whether I'll end up remaindering my cookbooks at a loss. I went on to reason that if I had put all my money into medical bills, I would have had no possibility whatsoever of a future income to pay other medical bills—not to mention rent, food, and subway fares. Frustrated, she finally said, "well, I'll have to get the manager."*

When she left me alone in this welfare environment with a disconnected phone and no hair, I began to imagine I was so poor they wouldn't give me any more chemotherapy. My financial planning suddenly didn't seem as reasonable to me as it usually had since my divorce. I began to wonder whether they'd put me in jail if I didn't come up with $1,700. I started to get pretty scared and even considered running out of there and pretending I hadn't talked to her. But then I imagined Miss Duby and the manager bursting in to the chemo unit, pointing at me sitting innocently with no hair in a chemo station, a drip taped to the back of my hand, talking to the nurse as if nothing were wrong, shouting for all the other chemo patients in the unit to hear, "There she is! She's the one who won't pay."

I was a total wreck by the time the manager swept through the door and said, "Hello, Ms. Mitchell, I'm Tom Watson." I pulled myself together enough to reply, "<u>The</u> Tom Watson, of IBM?" He laughed and said he wished he were. Then he told me that two months ago they started a new program at Sloan-Kettering for people who don't get Medicaid and whose insurance is not enough to cover their bills. (The only reason I don't qualify for Medicaid is that I've invested in my cookbook and have put $4,000 in an IRA that I can't get out until I'm fifty-nine.) I have the best insurance I can get, for an individual policy of a person who has had cancer.

Tom Watson commented, "if I were in this bleak a situation, I'd take off for Paris!" I responded, "I do!" He told me that he rents an apartment in Montmartre for a month every summer, right near Sacre Coeur. I almost couldn't believe it: that's where my apartment is too. The only difference is that I "house-sit" for mine and that he pays for his. He even drew a little map showing how close our apartments are. Back to the bill. He asked what I wanted to pay each month. I said $100. So he cheerfully wrote out our understanding. As he hurried out, Tom's friendly encouragement reminded me of Santa Claus's "And a Merry Christmas to all and to all a good night," as he called out to me, "If this hospital ever calls you and harasses you about money, you just tell them to call Tom Watson. And if you sell a book, you can pay more; if you don't, you can call me and pay less. You don't have a worry in the world!" Ahhhhh! Pure grace, undeserved help and protection was shining down on me.

So here I am, in the biggest city of all, and I've been offered a new program designed for people just like me. My surgeon had already said he would knock something off his bill, because he charges his patients assuming the insurance pays 80 percent. It looks like I won't go to jail or to the poor farm after all.

Now. To make some new money. I have a new plan besides the seven book projects I currently have out to thirty-five publishers. The plan is that I'm following my original business idea to bring out three cookbooks in three years. I've borrowed money for the next one: <u>Bread and Scripture on Wheels: Trailer Folks' Favorite Recipes, Chapter and Verse.</u> Christian-book sales have soared in the past two years, and the Christian-book stores have no cookbooks. That one will double my market from manufacturers of recreational vehicles. I am writing only quick-bread recipes (trailer folks still hate to cook and would never take the time for yeast breads), and there will be a line of Scripture on the bottom of each page celebrating the thrill of the great outdoors. It should be in production by May 1 for an October book.

So. I'm spending my days writing my cookbook in the morning, looking for apartments for Betsy in the afternoon, because she wants to buy instead of rent, and calling publishers in between.

I had lunch with Barbara Lucas yesterday, my editor from Harcourt for the disability books. You remember her; you cooked a New England boiled dinner when she came to Vermont to visit a few years ago. I had just finished a book with her when I got cancer the first time. Barbara is always so supportive and loving. She brought me a collector's 1930s map of Paris to cheer me up.

I bought a birthday tablecloth, napkins, favors, puzzles, and balloons to take to Ned. I plan to cook a birthday dinner for him in his apartment. I'm also taking him a red-and-white checked oilcloth, as he says they don't have a tablecloth. We are planning two nights in Yosemite. Won't that be wonderful? Maybe rent a bike for a day, or take a trail hike, which I'd like to do.

I'm going to Berkeley in the afternoon to see Freddy Behrens, Marge's son, who has cancer—a hopeless brain tumor. I've never met him, but we've heard of each other a lot. Marge has been out there twice. You can imagine how awful it is for her to see her son with such a discouraging prognosis. I get together with Marge almost once a week for dinner or something. Freddy has two teenagers at home, and this makes cancer in the family so much harder.

I'll be with Elizabeth on Saturday and Sunday, as we

start up California's spectacular Route 1 and stay just
north of Santa Barbara.
Back to my quick breads!

Love,
Joyce

Ned's going to be twenty! Before I knew my cancer had recurred, I had told him I'd come for his spring break. He wanted to go to Yosemite. I, like so many other parents with cancer, was eager to let my children see that living with cancer still means doing the things I planned and loved to do. Lita wanted to go too. She had never been to the West Coast and was very excited about a trip to Yosemite.

I decided to wear my wig to the airport. I put my red bandana in my pocket, deciding that I'd take my wig off once I got in my seat for that long flight. Not thinking too much of who was sitting beside me, I put my bandana on and, after moving my head this way and that, just took it off. I said something to the woman beside me about chemo, and she immediately responded that her mother had had cancer and chemotherapy. Then she asked if my twin sister had cancer as well. I couldn't imagine what she meant and said I didn't have a sister. She continued, "There was a woman by the check-in who looked exactly like you, only she had hair." It dawned on me that it was me in my wig. I reached into my backpack and pulled out my wig, and we both burst out laughing.

In Los Angeles, Elizabeth and a friend met us and drove us north toward Santa Cruz and Ned. We finally stopped at a motel at three o'clock in the morning, New York time. At last I got a chance to sit face to face with my daughter in the coffee shop. Sitting opposite Elizabeth, looking into her eyes, and learning her new perceptions of herself and the world was already worth the whole trip. She didn't ask me about cancer. She didn't talk about chemotherapy. It wasn't until a year later that I learned that she had been sure I was going to die this time around. It's almost an impossible task for teenagers who are working hard at their own developmental task of separating themselves from their family to support parents afflicted with cancer or undergoing any other crisis. Oftentimes the more scared they are, the less they say. Parents remain parents, and our teenagers are still our children—even when we have cancer.

Driving north the next morning, we arrived in Santa Cruz, where Ned had arranged for us to stay right on his spectacular campus, overlooking Monterey Bay, in the university's guest house in the middle of the redwoods. I can never get used to the "rural" look of California; I guess I always expected the whole state to be LA.

"Gee, Mom, you look like you've really been through a lot," Ned sounded so concerned.

"I do?"

"Yeah, I know you did awfully well . . ."

"My friends tell me how well I look."

"Yeah, I know everyone tells you how well you look, and I know you have a lot of courage but . . . but . . . you're my mom!"

Ned had found the best fish restaurant in town for dinner that night, knowing that I wasn't doing well on meat. He had even clipped for me a recent review of this wonderful small, homelike restaurant. As he ordered the wine, I enjoyed watching this grown-up young man and being in a social situation with him on his own territory. What a new experience for both of us! How proud I am of him! The next day I found Santa Cruz's best bakery and bought his birthday cake, then decorated his apartment with the balloons, party favors, and birthday tablecloth brought from the Big Apple. Ned, never a defensive guy with his parents, just relaxed and enjoyed it all. He invited about eight for dinner. Knowing that not many college kids cook lamb, I planned Ned's favorite, a leg of lamb, and it was a hit.

We left for Yosemite the next morning. The weather got colder and colder as we approached, but the air was very crisp and clear, the view tremendously beautiful. After a search, we finally located our cabin; it had two bedrooms and a little porch. It was idyllic, but for some reason, even in this spectacular environment, I was not feeling terribly well. I figured I was probably overtired. Ned wanted to cook out even though it was pitch-dark. So, using our flashlight, we found a campground and some firewood and started the fire under the grill to cook the steaks we had brought from Santa Cruz. We opened some wine, hoping it would warm us up in this cold but magnificent site. The black of the Yosemite ledges rose straight up all around us, so the sky looked as if we were seeing it from deep down inside an oval dipper, with coal-black sides. Every star shone above a very high horizon.

It must have been around thirty degrees the next day, when we cooked our breakfast of ham and eggs outdoors. This was the day to climb Yosemite. Waiting in the sun for a bus to take us to the foothills, I suddenly realized there was no way I could get up that wondrous mountain. Here I was, proving to Ned that chemotherapy didn't make any difference to my activities and life, and I could barely stand up. What was I thinking of? It would ruin the trip for Lita and Ned if I had to turn back halfway up. So I finally gave up and said, "I don't think I'm up to this. You go ahead, and I'll be in the cabin when you return. If you come back around two, we can have a late lunch." They assured me they'd hurry right back.

I hit the bed at nine-thirty in the morning, adding their blankets to my own, and didn't wake up until four. I felt nauseous, low on energy, and as if a sore throat were coming on—as miserable as anyone could feel in one of America's most spectacular outdoor wonders. What's wrong with me? Am I getting cancer again? Is the chemo not working? Oh, it couldn't be. I felt wonderful when I got cancer. I feel sick now.

It's four o'clock. Where are they? I was furious that they were that late. Then five, and dark, and then five-thirty. Fury turned to worry. Why haven't I called the rangers? What if something happens to them? Wouldn't they think it odd I waited until now to look for them? What on earth shall I do? Wait another five minutes. I hear someone now. . . . No, that's next door.

I was a complete wreck by five minutes before six, when I absolutely had to report them as missing and when up to the porch they came, their laughing voices full of the thrill of physical accomplishment. A six-pack of cold beer in his hands, "Oh, Mom, it was spectacular!" Ned and Lita had their beers and hot baths and were so high from their exhilarating climb that they hardly noticed that I wasn't going out to eat with them. My traveling pals had dinner in the Yosemite restaurant, where they had "hunter's stew" and a red California wine. It sounded perfect for them, even to sick me. By this time my priorities had changed: I wanted Ned to have a good time much more that I wanted to show him what it's like to be on chemo.

The next day we were on our way home. Ned took the bus back to Santa Cruz, and we headed for the airport in Los Angeles.

Once I was back in the weekly routine of chemo, and heading toward the finish line, the cumulative effect of this treatment was taking its toll on me: I feel very brave and courageous whenever I walk into the chemo unit. I swing my arms, stand straight, feel strong. But when I hear "Ooops, sorry, the needle went right through" or "We blew that vein" or "Guess I'll have to try another one," my courage instantly collapses with the vein. It just takes one slip of the needle. Nothing hurts, and yet I fall completely apart.

The worst happened with three slips. I was alone and just about crawled out of there. I was very aware that my kind of courage doesn't hold up with imperfections. Walking out of that chemo with lost courage, two blown veins, and chemo fright, I couldn't get my coat on. I'll never forget the experience I had struggling with my coat and eventually turning for help to a young black man pushing a broom. He put down his broom, stood facing me, and even buttoned my coat. Then he reached over and turned down my collar, as I used to do for my children. In that simple act of helping me with my coat, he gave me the nurturing I so needed. A few minutes later, when a woman gave me her seat on the bus, I realized what pathos I must be communicating. To think how thin my courage really is scares me. To think how total strangers fill my human needs thrills me.

The Home Stretch

❖❀❖

I met an old woman in the chemo unit whose fingers were gnarled at the joints; she told me it was from chemo. When I asked what chemo she was on, she didn't know. When I asked if she had shown her hands to her doctor, she said "No, it's very painful, but it shows that the chemo is working and cancer cells are being killed off."

Everywhere I looked, I saw or smelled pain and medicine. It was more and more difficult to take my Cytoxan each day. I was getting a general nausea all the time. Funny. I had thought that the last couple of weeks it would be exciting to know I was almost done. Instead, actually in the home stretch, I felt more tired, more sick, and wondered if it would ever end, even as I knew I was finally finishing my chemo program. I dreaded the needles: I thought, That nurse is going to mess this up; I just know it. The weekly finger stick was always a fright, even though it was on different fingers.

It became more and more difficult to find a vein on my hand that would hold up.

During these last weeks I began to wonder what would happen next. Where would the cancer go, how long would it take to get there once I stopped chemotherapy, and what would the symptoms be?

Trying harder to get out of myself, I wrote a lot of letters during April and May. I had written to Ned in response to his acceptance to a study program in France, though not in Paris, where he would have preferred to be. His experience reminded me of how people deal with the unexpected crisis of cancer: "Life is like that. You plan and hope for one thing, and then something different comes up. What you finally catch on to is that it isn't the place and person and job or school that makes the difference—it's what you do with what comes your way. How you respond to what you've got. How you live with 'what is.' Everything is interesting in life. Even having cancer. I'm always curious about what my body will do with these drugs, what my head will do with my body, how hard I have to work to overcome depression and my sense of having no control, how easy or how hard it is to laugh or have joy—regardless of cancer."

I wrote to my friend Judy, the only American I met in New Guinea and who turned out to own property thirty miles from our farm in Wolcott. When I moved to New York, I left her without a confidante who would drive from a back farm to a log cabin, even farther in the woods in the middle of January or in April's mud season. Often I left my car and walked the last mile up her unplowed hill, or a mile down my dirt road when it had been flooded from the thaw. Oh God! How these out-of-staters romanticize rural, isolated living. We would sit and talk into the night about our husbands and children while we burned our supper on the wood stove, so badly did we need our conversations.

Writing to Judy now, I told her how different life is in New

York City, even with cancer: "Three of us got together here two nights ago: Lynne, the ODN filmmaker, and a Canadian sculptor, Paul Hunter. Both are in their late twenties, and the three of us are working on a joke-book idea for second- and third-graders. I just loved the combination of people. I made French Canadian pea soup and johnnycake for the occasion. And tomorrow Carol Scheer is bringing two young men, nineteen-year-old college stopouts, computer freaks, to brainstorm educational software (paid!). I've told you about Carol—early thirties, sparkling eyes, runs in the New York Marathon. She was at Random House, and we were doing a great software project together on college choice until she was fired. She has since married her boyfriend and moved to Florida and now gets educational software projects from all over the country. I just never had those opportunities in Vermont—and I simply love it."

And I told Judy of cancer: "Cancer stuff is going okay, although last week I was in bed most of the time from Wednesday through Sunday. I went out for very short excursions. I seem to be very tired and have some nausea. Okay so far this week. Have so much planned; hope I can keep up. After my visit to Ned in California I had a virus that seemed to last and last. I was off chemo for three weeks. I will be so happy to be off these drugs, and away from the smell of Sloan-Kettering. When I go over there on Mondays, I smell the alcohol and whatever and start feeling sick and edgy as soon as I walk in. If anything goes wrong—as it did last week, when it took three sticks to get the drugs started—I just go over the edge. Makes me realize how close to the surface my so-called courage is. As I usually tell myself, it's no big deal. But when they don't get the vein right away, I crumble immediately. A woman gave me her seat on the bus after all that, so I must have looked as if I'd had it."

Everything was getting harder to take. I wasn't feeling well, putting that Cytoxan in my mouth each morning, losing feeling in my fingers. The smell of alcohol flagged the chemo to come. I know the end was near, but not here yet.

In late April I decided to go to church without my wig. Big decision. I had about one-eighth of an inch of hair all over. It was thick and looked good to me—up from nothing. Even though I was still on chemo drugs that had a possible side effect of hair loss, once I got off Adriamycin, the total-hair-loss drug, my hair started growing back. But compared to people without chemo? At first I thought I'd wait until May 1, but this seemed the time to do it. I'd been without my wig before: at Sloan-Kettering in the chemo unit, at the workshop for chemo patients, at home, in Vermont the time I was skiing, and at restaurants with close friends. Besides, I'd seen a few others with very short hair, though not quite this short, and no one had seemed to stare. Okay. Courage. Here goes.

I walked into Bible class before church. I had no sooner sat down than Otto, known as the dean of our church, one of the favorite old-timers, spoke up to say to the class, "I think we should require the ladies to wear name tags in this class so that when they get a new hairstyle, we'll know who they are." How I laughed! It didn't occur to me that anyone would assume that I'd choose to have my hair cut like this.

Others said to me, "I love your new haircut," "It looks good," "You look like a tennis ball," "Its very becoming." When sitting in church near another of the old-timers, I asked, "Dot, how do I look without my wig?" She responded, "Oh, is that what happened to you? I was thinking that I was brave to get the back of mine cut so short until I looked up and noticed that Joyce has gone quite a few steps further, and it's short all over!"

At the door when leaving church, I commented on something specific in the sermon, and the senior minister said to me, "Do you know what I think is marvelous? You are getting your hair back." In this great big church in great big New York City, the minister is aware of my chemotherapy and the struggles symbolized by hair. Thank you, God. I feel your presence. I know that you are with me through your children. Come cancer or cure, life or death, I am sure that I am not alone. Just think of all those horror stories you hear about being alone in New York City. Who would have dreamed that a Vermonter in New York City could find a caring community the first year here—just when she needed it most?

Well, going to church without my wig was worth it. But still, the energy it takes to risk the chance that life will be okay is exhausting. I no sooner step out and get a good response than I have to go right home and go to bed to rest up for the next test. One minute I'm trying to decide whether I should give it a try and go ahead, and I'm all smiles about the encouraging response. But the very next minute I find myself in bed with the sheet drawn up over my head, hoping to stay there for the rest of the day.

Now here comes a big one—a trip to Ohio to visit my oldest friend, Natalie, a retired professor at Denison, whom I've usually seen at least once a year. It was planned for late April, when her asparagus would have just barely come up, when it's warm. I can usually relax with Natalie: I can be quiet, read, work on my projects, and be with her friends, who have grown to be my friends too. All the professors I had in the 1950s are still there. To go to church and look up at the choir and see them all singing away in their seventies and eighties is quite an experience. Her friends had been following my progress with chemo.

Hair. What will she say and think? How will she respond? Will she wish I'd brought my wig to wear to church, to dinner with her friends? Will she get a kick out of my short hair and like it? Getting off the plane, I looked up to where the people were waiting for their visitors, spotted Natalie right in the front row, and waved to her. She didn't respond. I walked quickly toward her, but she looked right past me. Oh no! My

Natalie, who has known me as well as almost anybody for more than thirty years, doesn't even recognize me.

It's finally here. May 6. My last day of chemo. It doesn't feel as great as I thought it would. In fact, I'm exhausted just thinking of getting to Sloan-Kettering today. But still, it is the very last one.

May 6, 1985

Dear Mother,

Wishing you a happy Mother's Day on this happy day for me. Last chemo treatment. Such a relief. So glad to think of getting these poisons out of my system and getting back in shape again. To run. And not be sick all the time. To get my energy back. Not to mention my hair. I wear it "as is" now, and most people think I have a very expensive French cut. Parker is taking me to lunch today, just before my last chemo. That's typical of him: always there at crucial times. And yesterday Marge Behrens took me to Alice Tully Hall, at Lincoln Center, to a chamber music group. I always love being with Marge.

Have a Happy Mother's Day in Newport.

Love,
Joyce

Elizabeth's Mother's Day phone call and her response to the end of my chemo was food for thought, as children's responses so often are. I told her I was about to have my last chemo hit. She replied, "Mom, you mean it's the last chemotherapy you'll ever have? Forever?" I had to stop and think about my statement and qualify it for me as well as for Elizabeth. I had meant my last chemo for this bout of cancer. I hadn't even thought of the next time until she brought in that forever word. There's nothing like our children to keep us honest!

Now that the chemo ordeal was finally over, I wanted to check in with Dr. Hellman. Thinking he might give me some clues to look for, I asked him where I could expect cancer to go next and how I would know. I was a letter writer and knew how often he was tied up or out of town, so letters worked very well for what I needed to know. Here were my questions for the moment:

May 9, 1985

TO: Dr. Samuel Hellman

I had my last chemo on Monday. I played my first tennis of the year early Wednesday. Today (Thursday) I took my last Cytoxan and ran around the reservoir for the first time since I began chemo. Oh yes, In order to come out even (with the exercise), I threw two Cytoxans down the toilet—for a pseudo sense of control!

I am scheduled for a bone scan on May 21, and I see Dr. Minelli on June 5. There's another follow-up with Dr. Sockol on June 13.

Now what? It doesn't make sense to be going back to three doctors for follow-ups. What's everyone looking for? Can't I look myself? After all, I'm the one who found cancer both times. I wonder if you can tell me what to look for and if I can then make an appointment with you to check further. For example, I am clear about looking for a lump in my right breast and for anything unusual on the left side of my chest. But I am not at all clear about other symptoms in other parts of my body. I guess I'm most worried about bone cancer—or breast cancer in my bones, as someone said to me, although I don't understand the difference. And lung cancer. I have had a deep lung cough for the past two weeks. I'm sure when my white blood cells climb back up to where they belong—without the chemotherapy—the cough will go away, but I mean in the future. What can I look for and what can I expect?

My theory is that I will be symptom free for a few years and that my recurrent condition that was present the first time in my cancer, and not wiped out by radiation, will then present itself again. Do you think so? After all of this time and treatment, do I have a prognosis? I would like to know what it is.

Well, do let me know about follow-up and prognosis. My feeling is that I should see you for specific reasons that you explain to me, and skip the other two doctors unless they want to do some special test, other than the usual quick look for things I could do as well.

In the meantime, I look untouched by cancer. My spirits are better than my body. Everyone responds very positively to my very expensive-looking "French" haircut. I just hope that my hair coming back in as soon as I got off Adriamycin isn't an indication of what the cancer cells are doing.

Looking forward to seeing you.

Yours with hope,
Joyce

A celebration is needed here! A picnic—on Mother's Day, Sunday, May 12. I want to document the end of chemotherapy. I'll call Grace and see if she can come in from White Plains. Friends from way back, Grace and I were camp counselors in Maine for several summers together in the early 1950s. Although she never saw me down and out, she kept in close touch with me throughout my ordeal.

Not only did Grace come, but she brought the best dish of all, a curried chicken salad. Ann brought champagne, and lime seltzer for me; Betsy and Lita brought fruit, cheese, salads, chips, and French bread. Ann-Marie, a French friend I met at the chemotherapy workshop, came too, even though she had a hit or more to go on her own chemotherapy program. She brought a very special goat's cheese that a French family makes in upstate New York.

Pure fun. We walked along Central Park's bridle path, circling the reservoir and over to the tennis courts. Every single one of us in the group was a tennis buff. We found a green, grassy knoll under the biggest oak tree, overlooking the courts. The tablecloth was laid, the blanket put down, the champagne and seltzer poured. Boy, did it feel good to be sitting on a blanket at this picnic with my friends for this marvelous occasion. Chemo is over: Hallelujah!

Betsy stood up and toasted, "To Joyce, who has fought the hard fight and WON THE CHEMO BATTLE!" Thrilled, I accepted all toasts. I had been so excited about the end of chemo—no more Cytoxan to keep me in a constant low-grade nausea—and so excited about this picnic with my friends that I hadn't taken in the fact that the battle was over and that I had indeed won. This celebration symbolized for me the loving support system that I had all along in my fight with chemo. It was easy for me to stand and raise my glass in thanksgiving "To my loving friends, who always cheered me on in my fight."

A few day's later I had a reply from Dr. Hellman.

May 17, 1985

Dear Joyce,

I am pleased that you are doing well. You are asking all the right questions. Unfortunately, they are difficult to answer in a letter. I believe you should be followed by one person and that person should see you at regular intervals. I do not believe that you can be responsible for

*your own care and for deciding when to see the doctor. I
believe that any one of us can act as that primary
physician. I suspect that Dr. Minelli might be the best
choice both because of his availability and because if you
are unlucky enough to get a recurrence, it is likely that he
will be most involved in its treatment.*

*It is difficult to answer you concerning symptoms.
Recurrence can occur as spread from the breast to bone,
liver, or lung. Any of these have different symptoms: for
bone it is usually significant pain; for lung it is cough or
shortness of breath. While you can monitor these to
some extent, as I said before, it is useful for you to be
seen by one of us. I appreciate your concern about costs.
You need to remind us of this each time you see us so
that we keep our tests to the bare minimum.*

Best wishes for continued recovery.

*Sincerely yours,
Sam*

Besides his letter, I learned from my second bout with
cancer never to say never. The mammogram question came
up again with Dr. Sockol, my surgeon. After hearing my
usual response, he quickly dismissed my theory that mammograms aren't worth the money, because they don't work
on me. "Win a few, lose a few," he said. "They're not 100
percent accurate, but for someone in your high-risk category,
who has had recurrent breast cancer, once a year is an
absolutely essential requirement." Of course, he's right. After
all, just because I get a book turned down twice, I'm not
persuaded not to try again. I remembered how much I value
persistence, and thought more about the mammogram
question. I found out that the National Cancer Institute
recommends that if a woman is between thirty-five and forty

years old, she should get a baseline for her record. That means having an X ray of her breast in a normal condition to contrast with possible symptoms later in life. After forty, a mammogram is recommended every year or two, and once a year after fifty. Those suggestions are for normal women, with no history of breast cancer, just ordinary risk. High-risk women like me, with recurrent cancer, are expected to have a test more often. With that in mind, I quietly signed up for my over-fifty, once-a-year mammogram.

No sooner had I finished my chemotherapy than I was sure I had bone cancer.

May 19, 1985

Dear Bill,

I was at the most wonderful Carnegie concert this afternoon, Beethoven's Ninth with over 120 in the chorus. It was the last of the season in our Sunday afternoon series. Most of them I missed because of chemo, but I loved the ones I got to. I knew the program, but not until I arrived and heard the music did I remember the fantastic sound and our excitement the time we drove into Boston, in the middle of the night, with the Ninth blasting on your tape.

I am writing to tell you that I'm really scared. And I have been for several days. I am not calling, because writing will help and because by the time you get this, I will know my situation. I had told you that when chemo was over, last week, I couldn't wait to get in shape and started jogging around the reservoir and playing tennis. I was a bit stiff, so I cut back drastically, just barely moving around the reservoir on Tuesday. On Wednesday my left leg hurt so much that I didn't do anything. By Wednesday night my left leg hurt a lot, and I said to Betsy, "it's foolish, but all of a sudden I thought this had better be a pulled muscle—and not bone cancer." We looked up pulled muscles, shin splints, and so on, and I didn't think any more about it until Friday, when I went out to New Jersey to visit Barbara Lucas for the weekend. When I got there, I found a big lump right on my shinbone, and I can hear a creaking sound when I bend my foot. She thinks I have a fracture. But why would I have a fracture? I didn't hit it, and it's not black and blue, yet it feels like a fracture (I've never had one, but I've never had anything that feels like this). The only reason I would have a fracture is if it is bone cancer.

Oh dear! Having raised that possibility, I can think only about how I've planned to have two to three years symptom free. In fact, until Friday it never occurred to me that I would not be symptom free for two to three years. I'm not prepared to deal with bone cancer now. I want to exercise, to run, and to play tennis. In the worst way.

Anyway. Will call Dr. Hellman first thing tomorrow morning (Monday) and Dr. Minelli if he isn't in. I'm quite sure if I describe all of this, they will know what it is. I'm scheduled for a bone scan on Tuesday afternoon, but now I worry about a broken bone, a muscle problem. Will it show up? Will cancer show up? Oh God! I can't really believe that would happen to me, but it's hard to think what else could make my leg so painful. I walked to church this morning, a very short distance, three blocks across town, and it was very painful. Each day since Wednesday has been a little worse.

Betsy is in Vermont this weekend for her daughter's graduation from UVM; I imagine you are there too. It's very unusual for me to be alone. I am finishing my last draft of the first chapter of my cancer book, and the next-to-last draft of my truck book. Have worked hard all weekend, as my goal is to get each of them to the publisher before I come to Vermont. I just hope I can come to Vermont, can go on the tennis court, and can walk some around Montreal on Friday—something I've planned to do for such a long time.

I called Marge after church—I always feel better when I talk with her. I just wanted to say out loud that I'm worried and scared. And that I don't want this to happen to me at all!

More later, love now.

I soon learned that it wasn't bone cancer, after all. Probably a pulled muscle along with oncoming joint problems from the chemo. Still, May and June were tough months, filled with worrying now about cancer and about money, about selling book ideas and about getting a job.

Other chemo patients who have gone through the chemotherapy program will probably agree that when the medication stops, it takes us a couple of months to get stabilized and confident that we are going to live a little longer. Everyone keeps asking us how we feel, and how we are, and what the latest doctor's report is. People don't dare mention their own cold, flu, or sprained ankle, as if those things didn't need our sympathy, because we've had cancer. The home stretch in chemo means getting back to our friends and family and their daily concerns. After all the attention we've been getting with cancer, getting beyond ourselves takes some adjusting that most of us haven't thought much about. Not quite able to let go of the notion of possible symptoms, I found in the next few months little relief in the worry department.

After Chemo

◇❀◇

I wonder if crossing the ocean makes everybody feel as carefree as it does me. There's something about going to Europe—about flying six hours and being in a different time zone by another six hours, about having an apartment in Paris that isn't "real world" to me. It's the place where I can go and the worries about cancer or symptoms, or about money or job or relationships, just fade away. The excitement of learning French, seeing family and friends in a different culture, and walking in the beauty of that spectacular city takes over.

The summer of 1985 in Paris was better than ever. First of all, Ned was in France after his junior year spent at the University of Poitiers and in Paris. Second, my favorite aunt Eunice decided that this was the year she would make her first trip to Paris. She was bringing her daughter, my cousin

Mary, with her. Kay and Annette, childhood Hardwick friends, wanted to come too—Annette after her eighteen months of chemo. And Marylynn finally decided that if her kids could afford to travel, why shouldn't she? My brother John wasn't far away, teaching at America's NATO base in Holland, and planned to spend at least a week with our Hardwick family and friends. Because he lives in Europe, I can never get enough of my younger brother. Third, I had dreamed about my Paris apartment all winter long, during those chemo bouts, and often decided that I'd never be well enough to go again.

With the best apartment yet, right below Sacre Coeur, and everybody chipping in for the rent, I figured it would have cost more to stay home. At one time there were eight Vermonters together in Paris and six from our little Vermont village of twelve hundred. It was a very happy summer, marked by great relief from worries about cancer symptoms.

I got back just in time to spend Labor Day on the beach. I woke up the next day with with an odd-looking skin condition on my nose. Even though chemo patients try hard to feel symptom free, they have to do something when physical symptoms appear. I didn't want to call a doctor. I waited until what looked like poison ivy covering the bridge of my nose swelled so much that my eyes disappeared; the alcohol I dabbed on my nose, as instructed by my first-aid book, dripped into my closed eyes; the oozing clogged my nose during the hottest night of the year; and what looked like little patches of poison ivy erupted on my left hand (the one without lymph nodes and immunity) as well as on my right side.

I talked to Betsy about calling a doctor, and she concurred. But whom to call? Here in New York City every doctor is a specialist within a specialty. Even if I had the name of a generalist, I wouldn't take my oozing nose and skin to just anybody. I thought of all the drugs a regular doctor would give me, starting with Prednisone, and wondered what that could do to my sleeping cancer cells. Then I began to wonder if there is some special kind of skin cancer that looks like poison ivy that I don't know about—yet.

Maybe I should call Dr. Minelli's office the first thing on Thursday morning. After all, he'll know which drugs are compatible for anyone who's just been on chemo. And if I start talking about it, and it sounds like that special skin cancer I don't know about, he'll tell me to rush right in there and he'll have a look at it and tell me the bad news.

Finally, I decided to call Dr. Hellman's office. He could surely direct me to special skin doctors at Sloan-Kettering. That place has dietitians and dentists especially for cancer patients; it must have special skin doctors as well. Besides, little, lively Lisa, his receptionist, has speedy answers to everything and is always so cheerful about them. True, she talks so fast I can hardly understand her, but she's certainly the person to start with.

Little, lively Lisa. Don't you just have to smile when you think of this solid bundle of high energy, not five feet tall, with the deepest brown eyes, which sparkle so much you think they must be plugged into something, working in the very serious office of the physician in chief of the cancer center of the world? It just shows you what a sense of humor Dr. Hellman has. Maybe she's his niece, and his sister said to him, "Sam, no one will hire Lisa; she makes everyone else around her feel so lazy. Can't you find something for her to do over there at Sloan-Kettering with you?" Wanting to help out his sister, he may have replied, "Sure, I'll give Lisa a try here with me." Or maybe he thought contrasts are what make life exciting. The most lively person around a life-threatening cancer center would provide that contrast. I don't know how she got there. I do know that she always wears jeans or cords, with a bright-colored sweater and Reeboks, and always sits on the edge of a rolling chair, off to the right or left of the chair, never on the center edge, like most edge-of-the-chair sitters. She has several phones, envelopes to do something with piled high on her desk, at least three other people in front of her desk, another walking from an office behind her, and someone new coming in the door. She's always in the tennis "ready position," prepared to pounce from that rolling chair, footwork like a dancing boxer's, eyes searching the target for that return of serve— hard, even when it's lobbed over. And then—BAM!come the rapid replies to everyone's questions. If you're right there in front of her and can read lips, you're ahead of the game, because you can use your eyes and ears—everything you've got—to catch her return.

That particular morning I was not there when I reached Lisa at 8:45. I had to depend solely on my ears. Giving her my full attention and concentration, I listened while she said that between patients she was working on a hundred press releases this morning. I could picture her licking those envelopes while someone hesitated before requesting something. It was the perfect job for Lisa: stuffing envelopes to use up that high energy while others were drawing a breath. Sure enough, I hardly got the problem out—"an extreme case of something that looks like poison ivy . . ."—and as fast as any human being can say it, she said, "SurecutieseeDrGalli5737287."

"Wait a minute, Lisa, what's his name?"

"Galli5737287."

Pencil in hand, I felt like an old Vermonter when trying to listen to Lisa. She gave me the name one more time but then she must have decided I was much too incompetent to get an appointment if I couldn't even write down the name and number. Before I knew it, she shot back, "but I'll call for you, hon, because you'll need a referral. Are you going to be home?"

Lisa takes me back to the days of the height of the

women's movement, when I resented being called hon, always pointing out to Bill that he wasn't called hon, dearie, or sweetie, by receptionists, dentists, and clerks. Now, coming from little, lively Lisa, it was different. I soon learned that she doesn't discriminate at all. Everyone—even a robust, healthy white powerful man—gets called cutie by Lisa! If Lisa could get a special skin cancer doctor to look at my nose, which was afflicted with what was probably a rare kind of skin cancer, her diminutive names for me were pure balm on a wound.

I showed up for a one o'clock appointment in Sloan-Kettering's outpatient building, on the fourth floor—same as for chemo. I heard Dr. Minelli's voice booming at top volume over the loudspeaker as he called a patient, jolting everyone out of their inattention to what they were there for. I decided to go into the chemo unit and say hi to Connie. I got a hearty greeting in return, even though it was months since I'd been in.

Looking around, I saw the women with wigs, the friends of chemo patients, the anxiety on some of the faces, the tuned-out look on others. And, of course, those busy with their reading. What were those chemo patients thinking? What plan of action did they have in mind for coping with the side effects they would all be experiencing within the next twelve hours?

And now for the usual wait. I had taken a lot of work with me, but not more than three hours' worth. My nose was oozing so much that you couldn't make out its shape. It looked like open, wet, raw skin all out of shape. Others looked at me and quickly glanced away. This is how lepers must feel. Everyone sees the diseased condition—right on my nose—and thinks it's cancer.

I saw the doctor, who assured me in less than a minute that it was poison ivy, that I couldn't take Prednisone, the usual prescription for poison ivy, because I'd had breast cancer, but he was giving me an antibiotic plus a cream (cortisone) to heal it. The hospital pharmacy didn't have the cream, so I walked to the nearest drugstore, thinking the druggist would hit me for eight or ten dollars. I wasn't prepared when he said forty.

"Forty dollars? Never mind, I don't want it!" Tears started streaming down my face for the first time since I'd begun this poison ivy ordeal.

Surprised, he said, "But you need it . . ."

"Don't you have a smaller tube?"

Looking at the 60 cc's, he replied, "Yes, but its almost as much money."

I took it, then stood crying at the bus stop—mostly about my bad luck. I certainly don't need poison ivy, my nose oozing, my eyes swollen, and the doctor charging me seventy-five dollars for two minutes, at most, of his time. When I questioned him about the charge, he told me I didn't even have a regular appointment, or it would have been more. This was merely a consultation fee, and he was seeing me only to do Dr. Hellman a favor. So there.

Next day I woke up with a much worse condition, eyes swollen shut and nose oozing at peak. I was very relieved I didn't have to start today to find a doctor and, once there, drop over a hundred dollars on top of it all.

It's been two weeks. My nose looks okay. But the rash on my legs, my stomach, the back of my legs, and the palm of my left hand has driven me crazy at night. I just wake up scratching, and that huge tube is all gone. When Betsy asked me if I wanted her to pick up another tube of cortisone, I said absolutely not: "I've spent enough money on this itch. From now on it can take care of itself. My body can start on some immunity of its own, or I'll just make a paste from baking soda and water, or just itch. I've had it with nursing this disease; it's been pampered and medical-attentioned and creamed enough. It's the eighteenth of September and a long time since that Labor Day beach when I put the leaf on my nose to keep the sun away in the first place."

Now I just want to go to Vermont, see my mother and aunts, market my new cookbook, borrow Nancy's pickup to move some books to Bill's barn, play tennis with Bill, see Wewak, take my mother to my cousins to see the slides of our Paris trip, canoe on the Connecticut River with Judy, climb Mount Elmore to see the leaves, meet Hazel, and go to the new Hardwick restaurant. I don't want to stay there, but I do want to relax in my beautiful Vermont. As I said to Betsy, "My aunt Eunice will be so nice to me."

"Nice?"

"Yeah, she'll meet me at the plane, all excited to see me, drive me home, open a bottle of champagne, bake muffins in the morning, set a beautiful table with the best china, hurry around to be sure I have everything I want, hand me several new crisp ten-dollar bills in case I need more gas even though her brand-new car will have its tank filled and be equipped with her best Louis Armstrong tapes, and, finally, ask me where I want to meet for dinner after my cookbook work. PHEW. That's what I call being nice to me!"

I can't wait.

Skin cancer scare and poison ivy, good-bye. Vermont mountains, Hello.

Soon, back from Vermont, I was writing to Bill to say:

I've had a lot of problems since I've returned. My hands are very stiff; my thumbs don't work—catching at the joint when I try to bend them. I have to look at a finger joint and concentrate on bending it to get it to work. My knees are worse, and it's hard to believe but I can hardly step up into a bus. Can you imagine healthy me waiting for a kneeling bus! God! My self-image is sure off these days. (It reminds me of your response to a new haircut when we were first married: "It violates your self-image." I'd never heard of that before.) Even my hips are beginning to get stiff. It's all much worse when I first wake up and get out of bed, or get out of a chair.

I talked to Dr. Minelli on Monday and learned quite a few things. First of all, its not uncommon to get "joint problems" after chemo. No one had ever mentioned that before. Second, it's usually treated as arthritis. Third, he doesn't know if it will reverse itself and get better. That's a real blow. I figured all of this stiffness was a matter of my not yet having gotten back into shape from lack of exercise last year. Even worse, it can be an indication of more cancer. Needless to say, I am very discouraged. I am now scheduled for blood tests and a bone scan this Friday. Since learning all of this, I somehow feel exhausted and am much more stiff than last week, for example.

As you can imagine, all of my Christmas plans have to do with this rotten condition. I'm not sure if I'll be better or worse by then, but no matter how I go, I want to have something special to look forward to. This isn't to talk about with others. I just want to check things out and wait to see the best way to handle this joint problem. Betsy is a good sounding board, so I get quite an objective opinion from a health-oriented person when I discuss it with her and also when she sees how I move around the place.

Some of my friends thought it odd that I kept in such close touch with Bill over these issues. In fact, they said, from the way I carried on about how wonderful it was to be sharing an apartment with a friend, and how much better it was to communicate with Bill now that I was divorced, it sounded as if I preferred friendship to marriage! Good Lord. Is that the impression I give? I don't mean to. I think there is nothing more satisfying and fulfilling in this life than the joy of intimacy. Getting to know another human being in a trusting, intimate relationship that permits growth and demands commitment—has no substitute. When I first moved to New York City I thought, Wouldn't it be wonderful if Bill had wanted to move here too? Wouldn't he have loved this apartment? But then I remembered that's just fantasy. Bill doesn't want to be in New York; he wants to be on that farm. Even if it happened that Bill had moved back to New York, he would never have joined a church with me and have done all the things couples can do there—never spontaneously have invited people home for dinner, taken off at the last minute for standing room at the Metropolitan Opera with me, never taken a vacation with the children, or read my latest three-page book prospectus. Just as he didn't when we were married. The tough truth is that Bill never had time for me.

Intimacy isn't easy to arrange in our fifties. You don't get it by working for it, or by deserving it, or because you find it fascinating. Always being on the lookout for an intimate relationship brings a few false starts for any of us. And the disappointment that we haven't started on that second twenty-four-year relationship is something divorced people have to work out. On the other hand, those of us who have decided not to wait around until someone comes along to share our lives have endless possibilities with family and friends to give life our best shot. One of our possibilities is to be friends with our divorced spouse, the parent of our children.

Another bone scan was ordered because of my joint complaints. It was my second scan. Breast cancer patients get one before surgery. Dr. Sockol had told me that if my cancer had metastasized to my bones, it would be too late to remove the breast. I remember because he said, "It would be like closing the barn door after the horse had run away." I thought that a barn door was a funny image for a city doctor to be using.

I'll never forget that first bone scan. I found my way to nuclear medicine after winding all around in new places at Sloan-Kettering to a very lower-level, no-windows place, which looked like someone's cellar made into a waiting room. It was quite a contrast with the upper floors and their art, flowers, and windows looking out to the East River.

In this underground waiting room, with its stark, white-washed walls, there were only a line of straight chairs, a magazine rack, a water fountain, an oldish black man in whites with an employee's ID tag on his lapel asleep in a chair, and a white metal table. On the white metal table was a one-page handout that said, "Welcome to Nuclear Medicine." I thought it must be a joke. I mean, to a woman with college-age children who march in antinuclear demonstrations and talk antinuclear all the time, this welcome just seemed bizarre. It struck me so funny that I quickly looked up to the other waiting faces to see if they were smiling too. They weren't. I decided to take two extras to write letters to my children on the backs, so that they could learn what I knew about it. It turned out to be a very informative and helpful document, telling me exactly what, how, and when everything was going to happen. Well, almost. Here's what it said:

Welcome to Nuclear Medicine

While you are waiting, we are reading your chart to obtain a medical history which will help the physicians interpret your scan. We are also having your injection prepared for you. Each injection is made to order according to your approximate weight. The injection will be given to you in a vein and should hurt less than a blood test.

The injection you receive is a radioisotope. An isotope is a radioactive tracer material which will enable us to get "pictures" or "scans" of the area of interest. The amount of total body radiation is generally less than a chest x-ray. You will experience no sensations, reactions, allergic or side effects from this material.

For a *liver* scan, we request that you undress from the waist up and put on a white hospital gown. You will receive your injection and be asked to wait again for at least 15 minutes. It takes this long for the material to get to your liver and spleen so that we can get the pictures. We take several different views which take less than a half hour. To assist in landmarking for the scan, one of our doctors or nurses will examine your abdomen.

For a *bone* scan, you will receive your injection about two hours prior to scanning. You need not change from your regular clothing. You may leave the department after your injection. During this time, you may eat, drink, take medication, have other tests or take a stroll. If you are an in-patient, you will be brought back to your room for the two hours. It is helpful, however, to drink an extra 2 glasses of liquids (anything: water, tea, juice, etc.) before returning for your bone scan. We will also ask you to empty your bladder immediately before your scan is started. Please be sure to report back to the reception desk promptly at your appointed return time. The scan itself will take about 30 minutes. You will be lying down and the scanner does not touch you while it prints out pictures for us. Most people find this very boring and often fall asleep.

When your scan is finished, please return to the waiting area until your scan is developed and your technician tells you that you can leave. The results of your test will be sent to the physician who ordered it.

We do many other types of scans. There are doctors, technicians and a nurse available to explain your test to you and answer your questions. Please do not hesitate to ask for help. We are here to make your stay in Nuclear Medicine as pleasant as possible.

What do chemo patients think a bone scan will be like? Many of us have seen them on the TV news, but we see only the close-up. So many technical things in medicine are frightening until we know what to expect. I'll never forget my imagination running away with me on the first time around. I ended up in a very cold place that didn't seem like a room. More like a stage set or a TV set with cameras all around. The walls and ceiling and doors all seemed to be movable, and scaffolding was all over the place. After getting on one of the many tables, I noticed a big monitor in the room; several people were getting a scan at the same time. I could see the lights flashing and for some reason, the first time around, was under the impression that if I had bone cancer, the lights would flash at the monitor and an alarm would go off; but, of course, I wouldn't know which person in the room had the bone cancer! It turned out that I was wrong: you don't find out the test results for a few days, and then it has to be through your doctor. As the "Welcome to Nuclear Medicine" document points out, the attending technician or X-ray doctor doesn't tell you your results.

But before encountering the cold room and heavy metal, I got the shot that put in my veins the nuclear dye (radiation) that is later read by the machine. A doctor gives the injection. I said to the young man, "My veins look good, but I have learned since chemo that they aren't as good as they look, and you have to be careful not to go through them." "Oh," he said, "there's nothing to worry about here; you've got lots of good veins," as he proceeded to go right through that wonderful-looking vein.

"Sorry! Your veins are really fragile; they don't hold up as well as they look."

"Oh sure, it's not my veins that are the problem. It's that you decided you knew more about my veins than I did!" He looked at me in disbelief: Is this a patient talking to me like this? his body language told me.

God! There goes my courage again. The slip of the needle does it every time.

What if the radiation goes somewhere else? Not in the vein? Why is everything with a needle such a hassle? Why don't these young doctors let the nurses teach them how to draw blood or give a shot? No apology, just the same old, something's-wrong-with-you-when I-mess-up-with-this needle attitude.

Finally "the dye is cast," and I'm on my way to wait an hour or two.

Once I was on the table, the huge metal disk was put so close to my face that I was sure even my short nose would get crushed. Then I wondered what would happen if this huge, heavy metal machine fell on me. It's so close! Has anyone ever had anything bigger and heavier as close to his or her face as this? And been told not to move a muscle? What on earth do claustrophobic people do?

It's done, and I get the technician to tell me what he sees. With my X rays in his hand, he says, "No, the bone scan is clear of cancer. But . . . you have a joint disease in every joint in your body."

His words caused these questions to race through my head: Is that from the chemo? How much worse will it get? Will it stop? Will it reverse itself? Will it make my joints vulnerable, so cancer will go there next? Should I exercise more? Less? How have others handled it?

I made an appointment to see Dr. Hellman as soon as I could to ask him about my joints. What next?

I heard from a friend I'd been out of touch with for a while. I first met Jane Root at the Hyde Park Congregational Church in Vermont, where we were both members, but I'd heard about her way before we finally met and became crazy about each other. Jane had just retired from college teaching. Not one to do anything traditional, she and her husband sold their home and took off for the Peace Corps rather than settle in retirement as you're "supposed to." Jane and I had many entrepreneurial projects in the works: books, a TV series, and a consulting business on our "Learning on the Homefront" idea. Nothing ever got wholly off the ground, but it almost did. A film company wrote a treatment, and ABC was interested in us. We wrote scripts, acted our parts, sang the music, and even had the big-time meetings in New York two or three times. We both love children, are very traditional in what we expect from parents, and have a lot of things to say to help the family. Besides that, she has six children and I don't remember how many grandchildren. Oh yes! Another idea we had was to sell cassettes, with Jane reading good books to grandchildren.

The "joint" parts of my letter to Jane went like this:

I've had joint problems since getting back from Paris and have just started finding out what's wrong this week. It began in May, but I thought it was a matter of not getting "back into shape." I am always very stiff after running or tennis, or even after walking any distance. Then my thumb started getting locked into place, and I have to reach over and unlock it. Can you imagine? Then came the other thumb and my fingers; and my knees are especially bad, as are my feet. I finally called Dr. Minelli and had a bone scan last week. I found out Wednesday that it definitely is not cancer, but every single joint is involved and has an arthritis-like disease. They have no idea what that disease is. When they don't know, I think they should call it a "condition," rather than a "disease," don't you? After all, if they don't know what it is, how do they know it's a disease? And wouldn't you rather have an unknown "condition" than an unknown "disease"? I would!

Dr. Minelli said he'd never had a patient respond to chemo in this way before. As he is a young man, that's not surprising, so I said, "Well, let's talk to Dr. Hellman. He's been around a little longer and has heard of more things." The plan is do to a "workup" with X rays, and a blood test, and then to consult with a rheumatologist.

Now that I've told you all of that, Jane, let me say what this means to me. I'm glad to know it's not a matter of getting into shape, and no wonder my feet hurt after I run and I'm stiff after tennis. I now feel free to walk around stiff in the morning when I get up. Betsy and I had a good laugh about that the first day after the diagnosis. I am not going to focus on it. The doctors can get into working it up and diagnosis, but I really don't care as long as it's not cancer. I do play tennis and am stiff the next day—but the game is worth the stiffness. I wonder if this will make a certain joint vulnerable to the cancer, creating a good place for it to be if it's looking? Who knows? My energy is no different.

Selling books is increasingly harder for authors, because a few publishing companies are caught up in all these mergers, like the rest of the corporate world. Now if an editor likes a book, the idea has to go through so many editorial board meetings to seek a consensus for a big group of people. Authors also have their book ideas go through several editorial boards to sell one idea. My Making More Money, for retirees, has just been bought by Prentice Hall Press which is now owned by Simon and Schuster. Each time the editor called me to say,

"They like it," I thought it was sold. "Oh no," she said, "now it goes to the next editorial meeting and then to the president." Gone are the days when an editor at Dell said to me, "I like it," and started negotiating that minute for the contract.

Until I sell enough books to give me enough advances to even start paying a little each month on these doctor's bills, I am concentrating on finding a job. I've sent out about eighteen résumés in the past month and gotten one form letter back, and yesterday the first personal letter. So that's not a given, either. But I think it's only a matter of time. After all, I'm the one who writes books about how to get a job! If I can't do what I write, who can? I plan to finish my College Board book by Christmas. I'm keynoting for the state of Maryland for disabled young women and their parents. Two of my career books will be featured. Being with physically disabled teenagers will certainly help me get my mind off myself. In fact, my having had cancer and no hair will be an advantage to me in communicating with them.

I'm seriously thinking of going to Australia right after Christmas for three weeks, including one week in New Zealand. That was my plan last year when I was in the hospital—or the first part of my three-year survival plan. Now that I'm symptom free, I'm sure it's the time to go. I'd be with Lyn, and we'd visit all the New Zealand missionaries we knew in New Guinea. So if I get a job lined up now, I'll have the book, conference, and trip built into the conditions before I start; I won't be trying to negotiate all of that on a new job. The jobs I'm looking at are in writing, education, career development, and that kind of thing. I realize that there are lots of Ph.D.'s around who are going after these same jobs, so it may take a while longer than I had hoped to get something. My ideal job is director of college placement in an

outstanding educational community where I can be with
teenagers doing what I write most about.
                                        Thinking of you with love!
                                        Joyce

October 14, the day of my appointment with Dr. Hellman, finally arrived. I hurried into radiation, knowing how Dr. Hellman's unit would look, with a blackboard in the reception room on which were three or four names of patients to be seen by a group of other doctors who are always with him. Doctors in training, I always say. They come from all over the world, asking questions, reading charts, learning new things to take back to their own countries. It always feels so worthwhile (1) to be getting your own information, (2) to be an informant for others somewhere else, and (3) to be someone from whom others learn about cancer.

I had a short wait, not more than ten minutes, and then into the examination room came three very serious men: one from Israel, one from Central America, and Dr. Hellman. They were in their forties, obviously successful wherever they came from—all top dogs in oncology. They asked general questions, and I responded with something about my joints. After several more questions, the doctor from Israel asked if I'd been on Prednisone, and if I had gradually reduced it. I remembered kind of gradually reducing it, finally getting sick of it all, and throwing the last pills down the toilet. Then I wondered if the gradual part he was speaking about hadn't been gradual enough. I just couldn't remember how gradual the reduction was.

Dr. Hellman agreed with the other doctors that Prednisone, a steroid, probably caused the damage. He said, "Knowing that your financial picture isn't exactly a hit, I'd like you to try the poor man's (and woman's) solution. Rather than working it up at great expense with all kinds of tests, try two aspirin, three times a day, and you'll probably see the same results as you'd get from a rheumatologist's workup. At least try it for three months. I think the aspirin will eliminate the inflammation and the stiffness will go away." So. After discussing the effect of too much aspirin on the stomach, I bought coated aspirin on my way home and started right in.

In three months I would reevaluate the treatment and talk it over with Dr. Hellman and Dr. Minelli. For the first time since I was sure I had bone cancer, I felt good. I knew I'd had a thorough examination by three experienced, thinking doctors who considered everything in my case and came up with one reasonable way to go. After feeling so good about the day, I was very disappointed that night to feel my hands seeming to get worse. The following night I woke up with my knee bothering me for the first time while asleep. Just hold on. We'll see.

Two months and hundreds of aspirin later, I was truly out of the woods, symptom free, flying toward my darling daughter, Elizabeth, and eager for my first trip—to Australia—on my three-year survival plan.

December 19, 1985

Dear Sam,

My knees and feet are much better since I took six aspirin a day for about six weeks. My thumbs are the same. After my knees improved, I wondered whether, if I went off aspirin, they would stay improved, since I was no longer receiving the chemo that caused the problem. I have now been off aspirin for two weeks and increased my intake of vitamin C and calcium (for magic effect), and my knees remain the same. When I see Dr. Minelli in January, I'll see if he has any exercise ideas for my thumbs, but, medically speaking, I consider everything done that is essential.

In the meantime, I've turned in a 369-page manuscript,

the first book completed since this second bout with cancer. The book, <u>College to Career</u>, will be published by the College Board. I've also sold another career book to Prentice Hall, for retirees (who need $5,000 to $6,000 more a year for a quality life). But the biggest change for me is that I have a job. I will be directing a women's center in an inner-city college with the highest number of poor and minority students in the country. I kind of feel as if I'd joined the Peace Corps, or had a job in the Third World. It's perfect for me because even though it's low on money, it's high on freedom. I can take it in any direction I want to go, which will be mainly career development, bearing in mind that most women in the college already have young children to consider in their career needs and options.

But first, I am leaving for Australia and New Zealand to visit my missionary friends from New Guinea. You met one of them, Dr. Lyn Wark, who came to be with me in Boston for radiation. When she suggested coming to America to be with me for this recurrence, I said "No. if I am walking around next year at this time, I'll come see you." So, here I go on my three-year plan, made at Memorial last October: (1) Australia, (2) Israel, and (3) China.

You could say that I'm now working to support my cancer and travel habits.

I'm feeling so good, no loss of energy whatever. I know that cancer could still be progressing regardless of my energy level, but feeling good certainly makes for a quality life in the meantime.

I want to wish you the happiest of holidays, with many thanks for your medical judgment and tender, loving care.

Best love,
Joyce

Fight to Win!

◇✿◇

"**M**y doctor comes in and out of here so fast that it's impossible to ask him anything. Just his running in and out makes me forget the questions I was going to ask him anyway!" I remember the black woman in my exercise and talk-it-over class at Sloan-Kettering who said this to me. She was always crying. One day in class she told the group that she couldn't tell anyone at work where she was. She said when people go to the hospital they usually write their address on the bulletin board and everyone sends them cards or calls. But if you end up at Sloan-Kettering, everyone knows you have cancer, which, like leprosy, scares everyone off—they write you off as dead—you could lose your job—and in the meantime no support will be coming to her from the workplace.

I walked by this woman's room one morning and, peeking

in, found that she was still crying. A visiting friend was sitting by her bed, crying with her. I stepped in and asked if I could help. Knowing I asked millions of questions in class, she asked me how I got the doctor to answer my questions. Trying to get a smile out of her, I acted out a little scene. "First of all," I said, "write out all of your questions on a piece of paper before he gets here. Now, let's figure this out together. Let's start with your exercise rope over there. Get your friend to take your rope and stand right in back of this chair. Now, when the doctor comes running in here, you get his attention by smiling at him as if you didn't have any questions. Just as he relaxes, you jump out of bed and push him back in this chair, your friend will run around the back and quickly drop the rope around him and tie him there. Next, you relax, take out your list, and say, 'Listen here, Doc. I've got this list of questions. And we're going to stay right here until I understand everything on my list. So if you want to say it in a way nobody but a medic can understand, that's okay with me—I've got all week for you to figure out how to answer my questions until I understand.' "

The "control over the doctor" image soon had my tearful classmate and her friend in stitches. Then she shook her head and said, "I don't know how you do it. How can you be a fighter when you've got cancer?" I lowered my voice and whispered, "I'll tell you a secret: I was a fighter before I got cancer. Weren't you?"

"Yeah, but . . ."

Yeah but nothing! Think of your own history. Think of all those black women fighting for their lives. Think of Sojourner Truth, right on our U.S. postage stamps. They're all fighters. What's more important than fighting for your life? How else can we win our chemo battle, if we don't fight back? Isn't it only natural to fight for our lives? How much do we have to think about it? Are some of us so discouraged that fighting doesn't seem enough? So we sometimes think that our own personal fight isn't worth the effort to go up against this dreaded deadly disease? What more do we need to be encouraged enough to fight?

After all, we've read the stories about how cancer victims who have been pronounced as good as dead fight back, and the next thing you know the doctors are saying a miracle happened and the cancer is in remission. And we've read the scientific evidence that research shows that cancer patients who have a fighting spirit and who don't accept a negative verdict are far more likely to improve than those who stoically accept feelings of helplessness and hopelessness.

Let's say you agree. You do want to fight back. Then the big questions are, How can we fight cancer? How can we win? What does it mean to win the chemo battle? How can we win if our remission doesn't last? How can we win when we're dying? The first important step in winning the chemo battle is to accept the premise that winning doesn't mean living forever, or even living the normal range of years. Winning means the process of fighting for life in a life-threatening situation. As soon as we begin to fight, we take control; we change the quality of our life, regardless of whether we know where the cancer is or is not in our body. We take control by choosing to take action in our daily life with the sickness and the horrendous side effects of chemotherapy. We ask each other for ways to ease the side effects. We learn to notice when we feel well enough, even for part of a day, to rush in with our own agenda. We begin to recognize each moment that feels good enough for action. Our own agenda means exercise, our job, getting together with friends, reading, writing a letter, making a phone call—using our moment of energy to reach out to someone special, to acknowledge our encouraging friends. Taking advantage of the good moments of our life, that is the fight. Fighting gives us control, and control changes our condition of stress into a condition of healing. Going in the direction of rushing the good moments, however few, is winning.

Sound easy? Just get right in there and do what you most love to do—even as short as the time may be? There's a catch! You've got to know what you're going to do to make the most of your good moments. How to use the energy, for however short a time, to do what feels best for you. How to take over and not let the dreadful fact of cancer ruin the time you do have to enjoy life. After all, the answers aren't there for us with cancer. That's one of the most scary factors: there are so many unknowns. To think that even the front page of the *New York Times* in 1986 has to state, "Breast cancer continues to strike women with undiminished force and still baffles science. . . . What causes breast cancer and what can be done to prevent it—remains unanswered."

Those of you who have been through the treatment for cancer, or have been with friends and relatives who have, will have learned that you won't get every question answered, because there are no final answers. We won't get all the information we want, because it doesn't all exist, to make sound decisions or to feel on top of the situation. We won't get control by knowing everything, so we have to look somewhere else for control. That somewhere else has to be in the realm of what we do know. We do know how we feel right now. Take away the anxiety of not knowing, take away the fear of death, take away the dread of our disease, take away the guilty feeling for having cancer, take away the side effects of chemotherapy, and every single one of us has some time. Turning that time into actively seeking the good things in life—no matter how short—is where we can each find our personal answers and help our chemo family and friends find theirs.

I remember a Sunday afternoon when I looked out to a very blue sky. Sunday was always the day when I began to recover enough from a Thursday hit to think I was going to live until the next one. Finally stabilizing my stomach with part of a banana and my latest concoction of liquids, I thought about going out. A friend was visiting and asked if I felt like taking a little walk. I groaned but listened to what she had in mind. "On Ninetieth Street and Fifth Avenue, just a few blocks away, is a beautiful building, the National Academy of Design, and there's a fascinating show today of American landscapes," she said. "I think you'd love looking at those paintings; they're very much like those of the Hudson River School you liked at the National Gallery." I perked up, decided to give it a try, got dressed, walked slowly up the hill to Third Avenue, then up to Lexington and on to Park, and crossed Madison. There, on Fifth Avenue, was the loveliest-looking building I'd seen in a long time. The beauty of it thrilled me so. As I stood there taking it all in, I clearly remembered my first look at the Taj Mahal. Not that the buildings were the same, not that it was one of the wonders of the world, but my response was the same. That exhilarating experience of seeing a spectacular design in a building was the same. The wonder of a "something" that lifted me out of myself was the same. Once inside this very small gallery, I saw an exquisite winding staircase and chandelier that took me by surprise. I slowly walked up the elegant stairs, stopping often to gather my strength and to take in an art world—the most wonderful change from the medical world I could imagine. When I got back home, I looked at the clock and saw that I'd been gone for ninety minutes. I was astounded—all of that beauty and new perspective in just an hour and a half. It turned my life around. I knew that to be surprised by beauty was one important reason to live. It was worth side effects that I hate. Worth chemotherapy toward which I direct my anger, instead of cancer. Worth getting better for. Worth the fight.

Isn't it amazing that ninety minutes made the ordeal of

chemo worthwhile? What kind of an agenda can you bring to your life that shows the fight in you? Figuring out an agenda means we first have to figure out our values. In career development workshops for college students, I have often used an exercise to help them rank their values. I'd ask the students, "If you had one year, one month, one day to live, how would you live it?" I always used the question for students in the process of choosing their careers. I never thought I'd be living out that exercise because I had cancer. The lucky chemo patients have given their values and priorities some thought before they got cancer, before they started on chemo. Understanding ones values is hard for a lot of mothers who have spent most of their lives with shoulds about husband and children. Often, they don't see their own priorities, without the shoulds. It's not unusual for them to decide they should spend their time with their teenagers, or take a trip with their husband, when they really want to get away from the family or go visit their sister or a friend on their own. Mothers just aren't used to saying what they want. When they get cancer or a life-threatening disease is perhaps the first time that some women and men give themselves permission to ask, "What is my agenda?"

I met a woman in her early thirties at Sloan-Kettering who told me she had to be on chemo the rest of her life. Smiling, she said, "But I don't mind. I never knew my priorities until I got cancer, and I've turned my whole life around now, knowing what I want to do most and doing it. I think cancer is good for people. They get their priorities straight!" I was, to put it mildly, shocked, and I thought, Some of us with cancer already know our priorities. I had been through a divorce after twenty-four years of marriage and already had my priorities straight, and didn't need cancer to check them out.

I also met a man of about the same age who was told he had less than a year to live and who had no idea how he wanted to spend it. He had a young child and a wife whom he had been about to divorce before the diagnosis. He was sure he didn't want to be with them. He wasn't sure what he wanted to do. He gave up his work but missed it. He loved to play golf but didn't dare get out on the course, because he was afraid he'd have a seizure. Working out an agenda isn't automatic, as we can quickly see when we ask our friends, "How would you live your last year, month, day?" Now ask yourself, "How do I want to spend a one-, two-, or three-hour period of feeling better than usual? How will I fill my good moments? How will I make my life count, no matter how short?"

Another man, a well-known writer, has a wife who is dedicated to making the most of their time together, doing everything she can do to ensure that they have as many good moments as possible. When his cancer was first diagnosed, he was told he would never leave the hospital. By the time he had obtained a second opinion, he'd already had enough good moments to make him want to fight for his life. He and his wife take very slow walks to their favorite restaurants and often meet one friend there—any more than one is too many. "We usually have one course—a soup, or dessert and coffee, or small salad—and that's it," she says. "But it's the feeling of being where we like to be, for as short a time as it feels okay, that counts. Looking at him, most people think he doesn't have any 'good time,' but he does and so do I. We have freed ourselves from the consequences of what will happen next with cancer, and we do have thrilling moments of life, laughter, friendly faces—not just scared, worried, and feeling-sorry-for-us faces. At this point, we both consider our good times a miracle, each day we fight for his life."

One woman I talked to had a hard time saying no to all the people who wanted to come and visit her at home. Finally, she found an assertive way to say that a half hour with one friend when she felt up to it was how she wanted to spend her time. Knowing that she would see only whom she wanted to see within a time limit and that her friends understood, she began to enjoy her "up" time.

One's sense of time varies, from a few good minutes when we try to stabilize after a big hit to a couple of weeks before the next one. I decided to go for the big time—long weekends—if I ever recovered from the big hits. My first trip was in January to Key West, a perfect place for me. Without a single hair on my head: with that pale, white, sickly-looking scalp (very unlike the healthy tanned heads of men with naturally bald heads); without a prosthetic breast, because I hadn't been out of surgery for long, I fit right in with all the characters who roam the streets of Key West. I had a straw-hat but often went without it just to get a little sun. No one batted an eye, though. I swam in the pool in my T-shirt, but how I ever got myself seven miles out at sea on a snorkeling boat is beyond me. I was the one trying to stabilize her body. And I'm the one who always gets seasick, or carsick, or just any little motion sick. My friends had never been to Key West before and wanted to snorkel. Not until the boat kept going and going and going did I realize that we wouldn't be standing in the water; we'd be in water way over my five feet. That meant my life would depend on my swimming with my left arm. I looked around at the others on the boat with their snorkel and fins and suddenly noticed that they were all aged twenty, twenty-one, twenty-two, or twenty-five tops. I was the only single-breasted mother with fins on board. God! I thought. What am I doing here? I don't even care about looking at fish in an aquarium.

Not surprisingly, this exhausting experience had its consequences: my most dramatic cancer dream. I went to bed early, feeling low on energy and down after a day of too much sun, seasickness, and exercise. In my dream, I woke up, went into the bathroom, and looked into the mirror. My eyebrows had grown six to eight inches long, down over my face. I could see a small space on my forehead between where my hairline was supposed to be and this long, curly growth of eyebrow hair, which looked absolutely bizarre. I didn't know what to do: Should I cut them? Should I have a friend cut them? Should I call the doctor? Would they grow again if I cut them? My kids saw me, and at the same moment there was an automobile accident outside. A man had run over someone with a truck. I watched them pull the body out from under the truck; then everyone turned and looked at me and, seeing my weird eyebrows and no hair, started to chase me. I was in Vermont. It was winter, and the sidewalks were very icy. I had on my L. L. Bean boots but couldn't get enough traction to run fast. I tried to grab the rail at the iron bridge to pull me along and go faster and to get better traction. But it was too icy even with my good rubber tread. I started slipping and slipping. I could picture my boots trying to grab the ice, but it was no good; I couldn't get a firm hold and was helplessly slipping . . .

What a relief to wake up! What kinds of anxiety do we live with in our unconscious? How symbolic is hair, anyway? Maybe I wasn't getting away with looking like "one of the crowd" in Key West, after all.

My dream was just a dream. I knew what I was after in the real Key West. Having been there two years earlier without cancer, I knew what I wanted: eating fresh fish, having everything be within walking distance, reading on a beautiful beach, seeing tropical flowers and palms, seeing the sunset. It was all there. Being in warm, sunny Key West was wonderful; it gave me a real chance to recover, to gather my strength for the second phase.

And then there was that long Vermont ski weekend when the first big hits were all over. I was still on chemo, not drinking even a beer after skiing, but that Vermont weekend was nevertheless heavenly. I was testing again, wondering if my knees and legs would still work, wondering if my left arm would work. Could I push with my left ski pole? Carry my skis, poles, and boots to the lift? I was testing to see if life was still worth living. Testing to see if chemo was worth the agony. Testing to find out if I could really do my agenda.

I remember that Vermont friends who had heard about my chemotherapy ordeal expected me to look half-dead. So when they saw me in my ski clothes, they were surprised to see a person who was so healthy, ruddy, and vigorous—even without hair. Friendly Fidel, a Hardwick boy I grew up with, now the handsome man in charge of a Stowe chair lift, came running out of his little hut to give me a big kiss and say, "I heard you were skiing!" He just stood looking at me, nodding his head, eyes sparkling, and said, "I can't believe you're here." I could tell by Fidel's expressiveness that he, like others who knew me, changed his perception from "Poor Joyce, she's got cancer again," after they saw me.

Those were the good, big times in my chemo program. The shorter times were good, too. The walks, the letters, the phone calls, the oatmeal, the first thing that settled in my stomach, the new day without hyper smells, the forgetting that my body was loaded with poisons and the remembering that chemo was going after and killing those intrusive, unwanted, undeserved cancer cells. Looking at life rather than fearing death is what it's all about.

The trick is to know what you want, and to go after the smallest corner of that want: the most ordinary taste, smell, sight, sound, or touch of life. Clearing the mind of disappointments of the past, worries about the future, and fear of death is necessary before we can immerse ourselves in life. We can't enjoy the moment if we're hanging on to guilt, worrying what's going to become of us, and fearing that we won't be here for our next birthday or the children's next Christmas. Even when we have no idea if another good moment will come, we can still learn to ease out all thoughts of past nausea, of the blown vein, of the repugnant smells of the world storming into our nose through Cytoxan.

You can do it! I recovered from my last chemo hit enough to enjoy this perfectly baked potato. Crisp on the outside, steaming hot and soft enough to mash with butter on the inside, and that cool sour cream with chives dabbed in the middle. Now just hand me the burgundy pepper mill I found in Paris, and the memories of France come flooding in. Remember that upper-class neighborhood café, right near the Parc Monceau? The one with the two older ladies all dressed up and wearing lots of makeup and huge strawhats, their perfectly coiffed poodles sitting in their laps eating from the table too? Look, friends, . . . I'm winning.

Postscript

◇❀◇

Dear Ned and Elizabeth,

I've won the chemo battle! How do I know? Because
for the first time since October 1984 I'm worried about
my future. About doctors' bills, a job, selling book ideas,
insurance, friendships, IRA, time off, Saturday nights,
buying a co-op, meeting new people, and all of those
worries of life that are suddenly filling my mind. As I said
to Parker, "Now that I'm going to live, I've got to start
figuring out how to pay for it."

What's more, I've been feeling so well that I even
thought that I don't need a three-year symptom-free
travel plan anymore. Then when my knees started to give
me trouble, I decided I'd better go with my plan. It begins
with Lyn in Australia. We will go to New Zealand to see

*all of our missionary friends who introduced us to your
first-grade correspondence school from the deep bush of
New Guinea. I have decided that even if cancer survival
were not the issue, my three trips would be a good plan
anyway, for a single woman with a grown family.*

*It's so interesting to notice how far from ordinary daily
life persons can get when they're focusing on healing
from a life-threatening disease. I wonder if I'd get this far
removed from the real world—from bills and work
responsibilities—if I were healing from a broken leg or
appendicitis, for example. Any surgery not connected with
cancer seems so simple. All you have to do is get better
from the surgery. There are no worries about cancer cells
traveling around your body after you're healed. No
wondering where cancer might go or how long it would
take to find out. No interns and residents or new doctors
to remind me, when I ask what's next, "We just wait for
the symptoms."*

*And here I am symptom free for months. Even though
I was sure those first six months after chemotherapy that
I had bone cancer twice (shinsplints from running),
cancer on my nose once (poison ivy), lung cancer once (a
cold), cancer of the colon once (diarrhea), and a possible
brain tumor (tripped on the sidewalk) just about a month
ago.*

*Ordinary life challenges of what I want to do and how
I'll pay for it are a great relief. Now I feel that I'm out of
the cancer battle (death) and back to that exhilarating,
stimulating battle of daily living (life), where the
consequences aren't so grave—no matter how tough
things are at times.*

*And I'm so proud of my children and how they
handled having a mother with cancer, especially since
they were aware of the horrendous trial of chemotherapy.
I could see you both grow and gather strength right in*

front of me: from our visit in California and in New York City and from your letters and calls.

Well, Ned and Elizabeth, we've all learned from cancer. Lots about how many important things in life we have absolutely no control over. Like disease and weather and whom we fall in love with. I learned about those things for the first time in New Guinea. I remember Don McGregor, a New Zealand missionary, telling me that New Guinea brings everyone to his knees. It is also called a lesson in humility. I soon learned that regardless of skin color, level of education, career achievements, or money, everyone has the same problem crossing the flooding river. There is no privilege of birth, family, education, or money that helps you get where you want to go; there are no alternatives. You can't turn back and take another road, find a place in the river with a bridge, telephone, and say you're going to be late; you just have to wait for the river. Maybe a day, maybe two or three—no matter who you are. I hadn't thought of that in ten years, until this bout with cancer. So cancer, like a flood, reminds us of our limits.

Cancer also reminds me to tell the people I love that I love them. It reminds me, too, not to worry about the things I can't control and to do something about the things I can control. We do have control over many things, mostly over how we deal with the "uncontrollable." So figure out what you want and fight for it! If what you get falls short, the control you have is to make the best of "what is." And so let's agree to fight for what we want and to make the most of what we get.

I think I've got it pretty straight now. I feel I've been helped to number my days, and I'm all for appreciating life and the people in it. I want to start with you, Ned and Elizabeth, and to tell you today that I love each of you very much. I'm so proud of your questions and *decisions, and perspectives and openness to many ways to go in life. Thank you both for your extraordinary giving: I see it with me, and I see it with your many and varied friends as well.*

With so much love, hope, and admiration for you both,
Mom

Index

✧❀✧